The NEW PSY-COSMETOLOGIST

Donald W. Scoleri & Dr. Lewis E. Losoncy

A *SALON TODAY*
PUBLICATION

SALON TODAY
MANAGEMENT MAGAZINE
PEOPLE-MEDIA, INC, PUBLISHERS

343 Morgantown Road
Reading, PA 19603
(215) 376-0500
1-800-445-7789

4th Printing April 1990

Printed in the United States of America.

ISBN 0-9615591-0-1

A special discount is available on bulk quantities of this book. Contact People-Media, Inc., P. O. Box 91, Reading, PA 19603 (215) 376-0500.

TABLE OF CONTENTS

Tears streamed from her eyes as the well-dressed attorney clasped her attache case. In the heart of the Phoenix airport, the roar of 727s broke the silence. Neither of us co-authors dared to speak, knowing that she, as the stranger, had the privilege of resuming the conversation. Finally, the young businesswoman spoke.

When you two first started to speak, I thought that you were exaggerating, overstating the case. I mean, an operator, or what you call a psy-cosmetologist, being important in society? I thought, "What do they do but cut hair? Why the big deal?" And then as you talked about their far-reaching impact in the neighborhood, the community, even society, it really opened my eyes.

Another silence.

You see, my mother was an operator, and I guess I never had much respect for her job. But now I think of the calls she would get at night to help her customers, I mean clients, for their proms or weddings or whatever, and how she would put ribbons in the little girls' hair, including my own, to give that extra touch, that extra good feeling.

I never thought about it. I just took her for granted. And yet she has done more for people than I could ever do. I just wish I would have thought about these things before. I wish I could have communicated more respect for her.

To the cosmetologists and the barber-stylists who have touched nearly everyone's life, we would like to communicate our respect for you. We have learned from you, laughed with you, sung with you, cried with you, and watched you grow, watched your pride develop, and watched the world open its eyes and heart to you.

FOREWORD

Upon publication in 1985, *The New Psy-Cosmetologist* hit the beauty business like a thunderbolt. Here were two top salon consultants saying the future of our business depended more upon human relations skills than upon technical skills! It was revolutionary thinking.

Just one year later, the philosophy of *The New Psy-Cosmetologist* has been accepted—**embraced**—by thousands of salon professionals from coast to coast in the United States. The book's teachings have spread not only north to Canada, but even farther afield. When co-authors Donald Scoleri and Dr. Lewis Losoncy toured Australia and New Zealand not long ago, they received heroes' welcomes. The concept of psy-cosmetology has truly raised the status of the salon professional and enhanced the reputation of our industry as a whole.

So much has happened since that first printing! *The New Psy-Cosmetologist* School Program is now being added to innumerable curriculums, *The New Psy-Cosmetologist* In-Salon Program has been developed as an answer to the needs of salons who can't send their entire staffs to a seminar, and *The New Psy-Cosmetologist* Seminar and Workshops led by Donald Scoleri and Dr. Jerry E. Smith continue to spread the word at sold-out two-day educational seminars. Psy-cosmetology, recognized by *The Wall Street Journal* and *Cable News Network*, is no longer the wave of the future. **The future is here!**

From "How We Cut" To "Who We Are"

The first revolution to hit the salons was the precision haircutting revolution, one which resulted in better techniques and more dignity for stylists. **Psy-cosmetology was born of the second revolution in our industry, the current revolution taking place in salons all over the world.**

However, this revolution is different. Whereas the first revolution was a change in *how one cuts,* the current revolution is a change in *who one is.*

This revolution, the Human Revolution, focuses not on shears and combs and blow-dryers, but on the very person holding those tools. This Human Revolution addresses not just the head of a client, but the total physical, psychological, even spiritual person in the chair. The Human Revolution sees the "operator" as a *professional cosmetologist,* and the "10 o'clock appointment" as *a person with hopes, dreams, loves, goals, fears, and anxieties.* This new wave views the client as coming into the salon not just for a haircut, but also for courage, for hope and, indeed, for no less than a fuller taste of life.

We are seeing the humanization of an entire profession before our very eyes, and the excitement is that we will reap the benefits of it. Indeed, it is happening in response to society's needs.

The Marriage of Psychology and Cosmetology

How did it happen? The industry had many advocates of professional cosmetology stature who foresaw this human wave. One man who recognized the importance of humanizing the professional salon industry was not a cosmetologist, but a psychologist, a man who, since 1975, had been bringing his human relations expertise to the beauty industry.

Dr. Lewis Losoncy—known affectionately to thousands of hairstylists as "Dr. Lew"—understood the benefits of working to change the view of cosmetologists and barber-stylists and their perspective on the client. By combining his efforts with the complementary skills and talents of another expert, Dr. Losoncy set out to give a clearer perspective on the important influence cosmetologists and barber-stylists have on the lives of their clients.

Donald Scoleri was the man who could best get the point across the salon professionals all over the country. The most practical human communication and salon management expert in the industry, Donald was the natural choice as a partner.

Donald Scoleri's warm way with people and his grass-roots knowledge of everyday salon experiences have won him the hearts of his peers. He has worked at every level of the industry—from cleansing technician to stylist, to colorist, to salon manager-owner, and at both distribution and manufacturing levels. He is a national educational leader.

What a combination of people—Dr. Lew Losoncy, psychologist, author of numerous psychology books, who has lectured in dozens of professions, and Donald Scoleri, a cosmetologist who has lived his entire working life studying this profession—have put this revolutionary book together.

For the first time, the industry that touches the lives of millions of people each day is explored and exposed.

For a profession that plays such a powerful role in people's lives, the people in it are relatively unknown and taken for granted. *The New Psy-Cosmetologist* dramatically highlights the world's most touching profession, where it's going, and how it will significantly affect *you* and your life.

Howard Hafetz, President
Raylon Corporation

**Cosmetologists
and
Barber-Stylists
of the 1970s**

**Emphasis on
*HOW WE CUT***

**Psy-Cosmetologists
of the
21st Century**

**Emphasis on
*WHO WE ARE***

INTRODUCTION

Imagine for a few seconds an electrical map of the United States and Canada. Now turn on the electricity in your mind to simultaneously light 160,000 dots across your map. Let's call these lighted dots *beauty salons or barber shops.*

Next envision within each of these salon lights an average of four people. Then imagine that each of these four people sees about forty clients a week. Hold on, that's not quite true; the word *see* is an understatement. Let's strive for accuracy. What they actually do with those 26 million clients a week is *touch,* not just see. Wait! Even touch doesn't quite do justice to what is actually happening in these relationships. What is really going on is that **these two-thirds of a million people are influencing the appearances** of fellow human beings who are sitting in their hydraulic chairs.

And could it be that in some cases it goes even further than that? Could it be that some of those 26 million clients sitting in those chairs each week are actually feeling better about themselves and their lives? **Could it be that in some cases those clients are gaining a little more confidence, a little more courage, a little more hope during this hour or so?** Could it be that they are sharing things about their lives with this friend who touches them six to fifty times a year—more frequently than some people see such loved ones as their mothers and fathers?

What other profession in the world could make the claim of touching people on a regular basis for a period of years, while giving a life-charging gift of beauty and confidence? Doesn't it give you a permanent lift knowing that these 160,000 lighthouses are out there?

Did you ever see these facts before? We didn't!

We must be totally honest with you right up front. Before we took an in-depth look at the contributions of people in the professional salon industry, their power simply went over our heads. We, one of us a psychologist, one a cosmetologist, started our safari into this unique profession with the mission of helping

1

the people working in those lighted dots to serve their clientele more effectively. But, as we ventured into the rich, varied, and unexplored terrain of the profession, we became overwhelmed with what we experienced. In fact, on the Tuesday before Christmas of 1983, we almost turned back, convinced that no one would ever believe what was actually going on in these places of beauty that you see almost everywhere—from the crowded street corners of New York and Miami to the winding country roads of West Virginia, to the golden wheat fields of Kansas, to the gallant snow-peaked Rockies of Alberta, Canada, to the Great Northwest and the lively streets of San Francisco.

Encouraging each other, we knew that our pens had to write what our eyes saw. We needed to share with that part of the world that seeks awareness the fact that those two-thirds of a million people working in those 160,000 dots might be a source of power for a large segment of society. Our adventure revealed to us that what we were studying was possibly one of the most influential professions in the modern world. **In these human lighthouses are stationed a vast group of people who literally touch society at its very roots.**

This book is about our journey through the professions of cosmetology and barber-styling, and how they affect the client. As you will soon see, it is a huge industry, a huge profession in dramatic transition. **A major revolution is occurring in those lighthouses. The revolution is a human one, a literal transformation in self-image.** The "operators" are increasingly being seen for what they are—*cosmetologists* or *barber-stylists*. In the coming years, they will be known as psy-cosmetologists trained in communicating with people and understanding human behavior, as well as having the skills to confer cosmetic beauty.

Have you noticed that neighborhood barber shops and beauty parlors are turning into professional, quality service centers staffed with specialists in cutting, coloring, perming, plus skin, nail, and cosmetic care? Wait until you see what else you'll find in the twenty-first-century salons! The owners are gradually giving up their shears and turning to books to develop their expertise in business and people management.

We have tried to capture the new wave taking place in the professional salon industry. We have concluded that the ones who stand to gain the most from this twenty-first-century Human Revolution are the 26 million clients who go to those 160,000 lighthouses each week. We believe that, until now, the hundreds of thousands of salon professionals who make most of the public shine have been taken for granted.

For a few pages, we'd like to shine a little light on them!

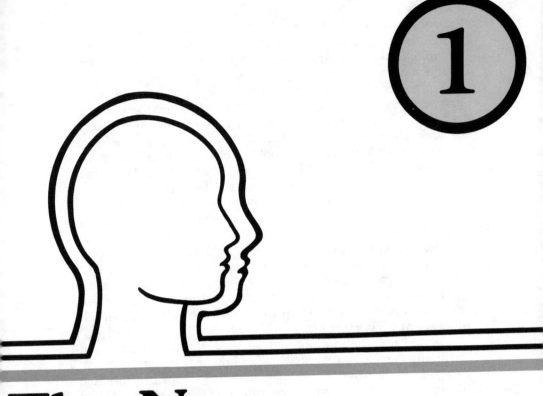

The New Psy-Cosmetologist's Special Relationship With The Client

Allow me to introduce myself first, and tell you how we co-authors met and why we wrote this book. My name is Lew Losoncy, and I was a counselor with a private practice in a downtown Reading, Pennsylvania office. At the same time, I was employed as a professor of psychology and was chairman of the department of behavioral science at the Reading Area Community College. A dramatic experience provided the impetus for me to learn more about the professions of cosmetology and barber-styling. Let me share with you the experience I had with one of my clients, Debbie, that caused such a change.

Debbie was an attractive, 22-year-old woman whose major problem, shyness, kept her from reaching her goal of getting a date with a local accountant named David. Oh, understand, she knew his patterns, the local lounges where he imbibed, and each Friday she would go to the Peanut Bar and R.J. Willoughby's to try to get close to the bespectacled bean counter, to no avail. He would totally ignore her and, frustrated, she would return to my "couch" to tell of her lack of progress with this "hunk".

After hearing the same old song week after week, I decided to encourage her to take a more assertive approach to fulfill her dreams of being with David.

Maybe David himself is shy, Debbie. Perhaps he too would like to go out with you, but just doesn't know how to go about it. I have a thought. Why don't you initiate a conversation with him, and if you two seem to click, you can ask him out for dinner?

What? You mean me just go up to him, she shivered, *and ask him out? A woman can't really do that, can she? I mean, wouldn't that be too pushy?*

Well, Deb, apparently what you are doing now isn't working, I replied. *At worst, he'll ignore you, and that's exactly where you are right now, isn't it? Imagine if you and David would really hit it off. No limits!*

A thoughtful, anxious silence filled the room, and soon the petite blonde lifted her chin with determination and replied, *Okay, Dr. Lew, I'm going to talk to David on Friday. I'm going to go right up to him and ask him to go out to dinner. That's that.*

She left the office with the determination of the ant who moved the rubber tree plant.

Did She or Didn't She?

My eagerness to hear the results of Debbie's plan made for a long week. When she arrived for her next appointment, I was surprised by her demeanor. Instead of an enthusiastic miss prancing into the room, in walked my client with a defeated, hang-dog expression. She slumped in her seat, and I had to ask her the big question.

Well, Deb, is there anything you'd like to tell me? I mean, did you talk to David on Friday?

Well, uh, no. I didn't, she timidly responded.

Oh? Can you tell me why you didn't follow through on our plan?

She replied with three sentences that changed my life! *Well, Doctor, I know you thought it would be a good idea to go up and talk to David. But, I talked to my hairdresser, and she thought it would be stupid. So I listened to her.*

I was never the same again! Despite my ten years of schooling and both a Master's and a Doctor's degree in counseling, Debbie trusted her hairdresser's advice more than she did mine!

How could a hairdresser be so important to a person? To answer that question, I decided to study the nature of that special relationship between the hairdresser and the client. But how could I get started?

GETTING MY HEAD IN THE SALON DOOR

Until this experience with Debbie, I had thought very infrequently about barbers and hairdressers. In fact, I cut my own hair. That started when my barber refused to give me, a teenager, anything but a crew cut, and I wanted to look like John Lennon. He was angry at long hair and told me to go elsewhere if I wanted to look like a freak. Also, he was so busy selling things like radios and jumper cables that cutting hair seemed secondary to him.

Being unfamiliar with the beauty or barbering professions, and having a deep desire to learn about the stylist/client relationship, I had to search through my list of friends to get me in the salon door.

A Little Help From My Friends

My parents had some wonderful, caring friends, Shirley and Eddie Weisburger. Besides being one of the most intelligent people I had ever met, Eddie was a vice president of a Pennsylvania-based beauty supply distributorship. This highly successful, young-thinking salon industry executive opened doors for me by asking me to address his sales force on communication and motivation.

It was at Eddie's company that I made contact with the legendary Joe Hafetz, President of the Raylon distributorship. Joe had helped build thousands of salons by educating and supplying products to the cosmetologists, barber-stylists, salon managers and owners of Pennsylvania, New Jersey, Delaware, Ohio, and West Virginia.

I was also privileged that day to meet Howard Hafetz, a far-thinking visionary who, at his young age, had already made dramatic contributions to the professional salon industry.* We had much in common—both of us knew that there was much more to a haircut than just a haircut. We talked for hours, burning the midnight oil about what a hairstylist really does. He supplied the opportunity for me to work with thousands of salon owners, managers, stylists, receptionists, cleansing technicians, and other specialists. I had my "in." The remarkable journey to the center of the stylist/client relationship had begun.

The Birth of Psy-Cosmetology

Howard told me about a man on the West Coast who was more in touch with the very heart, mind, and soul of the hairstylist than anyone he knew. He explained that this man, Donald Scoleri, was at the time lecturing throughout North America, obsessed with upgrading the skills and images of salon industry professionals.

In October of 1979, Howard conducted a program for stylists, owners, and managers. Donald and I were the two lecturers. Although we met for the first time that day, it felt like the reunion of two old friends. Our ideas, mine from the field of psychology and Donald's from the field of cosmetology, were in tune. The New Psy-Cosmetology was born. Howard Hafetz had arranged what could eventually lead to changed perceptions of over half-a-million members of a profession who have started to see themselves as they really are—the most influential profession in society at the grass-roots level.

This book is about the unbelievable insights we gained in our years of work within the professional salon industry. Howard

*Howard Hafetz was selected "Man Of The Year" in the professional salon industry in 1978 by MODERN SALON Magazine.

Hafetz' never-ending willingness to advise us, and to get us into salons in more than forty of the United States and in most of the Canadian provinces made this book happen.

What did we find?

THE UNIQUE RELATIONSHIP BETWEEN THE NEW PSY-COSMETOLOGIST AND THE CLIENT

Why did Debbie place such deep trust in her hairstylist? The more I visited and studied salons, the more I began to understand the important role cosmetologists and barber-stylists play in their clients' lives. **I discovered three primary reasons for the special and unique relationship between the cosmetologist or the barber-stylist and the client:**

Fact 1: **The cosmetologist is one of those rare professionals with a license to touch people.**

Fact 2: **The cosmetologist sees the client on a regular, ongoing basis, and before most of the client's major life events.**

Fact 3: **The cosmetologist has the power, the skills, and the tools to help the client look and feel more attractive, and in turn, more confident.**

Let's explore each of these facts separately . . .

FACT 1: The cosmetologist is one of those rare professionals with a license to touch people.

The cosmetologist does what the lawyer, the teacher, the accountant, and the chairman of the board don't dare to do. The cosmetologist *touches people.*

Touch is a vital need. The noted psychologist, Ashley Montagu, wrote in *Touching* of how we frequently use words relating to the sense of touch to describe everyday experiences. Touch is so important that it influences much of our thinking, even in our language. Montagu wrote:

We speak of rubbing people the wrong way . . . a soft touch . . . we get into touch or contact with others. Some people have to be handled carefully or with kid gloves. Some are thick skinned, some get under one's skin, while others remain only skin deep . . . Some people are touchy.

Some Die From Lack of Touch

Those who are touched tend to be healthier, warmer, and more emotionally stable people. Those who are not touched tend to be more aloof, cold, and suffering from emotional problems. In extreme cases, people *die* from lack of touch.

Two opposing kings in the Middle Ages were so grandiose that each believed his language to be *the* universal language and the language of the other king to be a fraud. They made a bet that, if young children were not talked to or touched, but just fed, the children would speak the true universal language, which each king believed would be his own language. They never found out which monarch was right, because all 24 infants died—not from lack of food, but from lack of *touch*.

In fact, half of the deaths in institutions in the early 1900s were due to cold treatment and lack of touch! The condition is called *marasmus* and is the result of insufficient personal contact.

The cosmetologist touches every client, every workday. The professional hair doctor is one of the few licensed professionals able to do so. But the hair designer's power of touch goes even further than that. **The cosmetologist may actually be healing diseases by fulfilling the client's important need for touch.**

Touch May Be Healing

The scientific writer, Charles Panati, wrote in his insightful book, *Breakthroughs*:

We realize that the human touch soothes, but it may also heal. In the future, doctors and nurses may be trained to hold their patients' hands or stroke their patients' injuries. In this way parents and children and spouses may to some extent become general physicians at home.

At the University of Maryland Medical School, Dr. James Lynch, a specialist in psychosomatic medicine, has found that petting animals has a beneficial effect on their cardiovascular systems; it also increases their resistance to infections. Similar results are being observed with human patients; even people in deep comas often register improved heart rate and brainwaves when their hands are held by doctors, nurses, or family members. Dr. Lynch extrapolates these early findings for a broad human base. There is a biological basis for our need to form human relationships. He says, "If we fail to fulfill that need, our health is in peril."

Although those biological foundations have yet to be discovered, one new medical treatment called therapeutic touch is gradually being introduced into hospitals and nursing schools around the country. Simply stated, nurses attempt to make sick patients feel better by a sort of "laying on of hands." Pioneered by Dr. Dolores Krieger of New York University's School of Nursing, the therapy creates a physical closeness between two people, even though the nurse never touches the patient but holds her hands about an inch above the patient's body (and not always the ailing part). Dr. Krieger suspects that the treating nurse actually transmits energy to the patient, which aids in recovery. Medical authorities are skeptical of that claim but agree that in many cases therapeutic touch works. Stroking a fevered forehead, holding the hand of a suffering patient, or merely sitting by a patient's bed—such a therapeutic touch may work simply because it raises the patient's spirits and, as a result, the bodily defenses. As holistic medicine teaches, anything that makes you feel better can also influence your recovery.

So far more than 3,000 doctors, nurses, therapists, and even some veterinarians have mastered the technique of therapeutic touch, and their number is steadily growing. More hospitals are permitting their staffs to practice the treatment as an adjunct to—never in place of—conventional therapies. Only future experiments will determine whether touching heals for physical or psychological reasons. In the meantime, we may see physicians in the 1980s and 1990s prescribing less medication and dispensing a lot more Tender Loving Care.

Think of it: the cosmetologist is licensed to touch each client, every workday. And the sad note is that **in some cases the hairstylist may be the only one who touches a client in his or her adult life!** This is especially troubling, because in today's technological society, people's need for touch is being even less fulfilled.

Our High Tech/High Touch Society

John Naisbitt, author of the powerful best-seller, *Megatrends*, advanced the strong argument that **the more technology exists in our world, the more people have a need for personal touch** (literal and figurative). Perhaps, in a way, the world is becoming less personal with the proliferation of computerization. People tend to feel more like things, like numbers, not like people. Most of us have a social security number, a license plate number, an insurance policy number, a credit card number, a telephone number, and an address number.

From our vantage point, **there is no place in communities of today and of the future that is in a better position to fill people's need for touch than in the salon,** with the warm touch of a stylist who knows our name. A stylist's everyday way of touching people, rarely realized, is a great factor in the special relationship with clients, and its importance goes beyond just a haircut. It fulfills one of the most basic human needs, the need for touch.

Shampooing: A Touching Experience

The shampooing done by a relaxed person who makes minimal demands on clients to think, talk, or answer questions can be anything from a relaxing to a sensual experience. Clients trust the cleansing technician enough to touch, in some cases, their dirty or dandruffed hair. And the cleansing technician accepts these clients without reprimand. Even their parents didn't do that! And so, trust begins to build.

No Strings Attached

Psychologists Stanley Standel and, later, Carl Rogers referred to a special relationship between two people as having the quality of *unconditional positive regard*. Unconditional positive regard is the feeling that exists in the best, most wholesome relationships. Unconditional positive regard communicates to the other, "I accept you with no conditions, no strings attached. You can feel safe to be you and express yourself without any pressure or fear of judgment. I have positive feelings for you based upon trust, you being you, even if your hair is not perfect." Couple unconditional positive regard with the relaxing shampooing experience and you begin to see the depth of the relationship that occurs in the shampooing setting.

Unmasking

In that touching setting, something else is occurring. **Cosmetologists are washing away their clients' masks, their psychological defenses.** A personal friend of ours, the well-known artist Charles Henry Norman, says that in a three-hour sitting with famous figures, giving them his sole attention and sketching in their facial details including blemishes, they tell him more about themselves than they have told some long-time friends. Norman explained: *You are addressing flaws about themselves head on that they are anxious about. And you still accept them. The contact is close.*

The cleansing technician, like the artist, is in charge, is benign, is accepting without conditions, and is interested. The client's fears, anxieties, and resistances are lowered. The client feels safe, even in an unprotected state. A shampoo would be the logical start of the therapeutic salon experience even if shampoos weren't necessary. It is the forerunner to the blossoming of beauty that is soon to occur.

Styling:
Touching To Remove Least Desirable Parts

The stylist wields a scissors, an aggressive weapon. From childhood, people have been cautioned to be careful when using knives and scissors. Yet **clients trust that the cosmetologist or barber-stylist will use this power tool to help them, not hurt them. They trust that the stylist will be discriminating enough to remove only those undesirable hairs of the head. They eagerly lift their heads at the stylist's will. For a period of time in their visit to the salon, they trust the stylist to see them at their worst, and he or she still accepts them.**

The relationship in some cases is so strong that many clients demand the individual attention of their stylists. Their annoyance while waiting in the reception area is many times related to the stylist's being with another client. Leaving a client to accept a personal phone call is often perceived as rejection, a statement that "something else is more important than me." Stylists have described clients who would ask them, "About how many people will you see today?" The question could certainly be a reflection of the feeling, "Am I just another customer to you?"

Along with the cosmetologist's license and ability to satisfy clients' needs for touch, a second reason for the powerful relationship is the frequency of contact.

FACT 2: The cosmetologist sees the client on a regular, ongoing basis, and before most of the client's major life events.

Delving into the nature of the relationship between hairdresser and client is, to say the least, an eye-opening experience. Yes, you find that hairdressers touch people. But the relationship goes much further than that. **Hairdressers see each client six to fifty times a year, sometimes over a period of twenty years or longer.** How many times a year do most of these clients see their relatives?

A survey published by *MODERN SALON Magazine* cited the following statistics in answer to the question, "How long have you been going to your current stylist?"

NUMBER OF YEARS	PERCENTAGE OF RESPONDENTS
More than 7	24.2%
7	5.4%
6	3.7%
5	10.5%
4	7.5%
3	12.6%
2	13.9%
1	8.3%
Less than 1	13.9%

By far, the largest category was more than seven years. **One out of four clients had been going to the same cosmetologist or barber-stylist for a period of longer than seven years.** Interestingly, male clients have even more stylist loyalty than female clients. And yet, so strong is the loyalty of female clients to their stylists that 93.7% go to the same stylist every time. Only 6.4% of the female respondents said that they would go to any stylist available.

Unlike the schoolteacher who is with a child for a period of only one year (on rare occasions, two years), and unlike the doctor who often sees a patient only once or twice a year for a checkup, **the professional hair designer is a regular in the client's life, sometimes even considered "family."** The lawyer is called in only in times of crisis. Dentists basically see patients every six months. Only the clergy/parishioner relationship is more frequent (once a week), but even that is not on a personal, one-to-one, touching basis.

The power of the psy-cosmetologist/client relationship goes beyond mere frequency. The cosmetologist is around people during family births, family deaths, and all emotionally provoking events in between.

A Haircut Is A Good Reason To Bring People Together Again

The public perception of what cosmetologists or barber-stylists do is that "they cut hair." If a stylist just cuts hair, why do the hair professionals we meet know most of their clients' husbands', wives', girlfriends', and boyfriends' names? In some cases, they know both the client's wife and the client's girlfriend! And in some communities, they cut the husband's, the wife's and the girlfriend's hair! As we said before, it is a *touchy* business!

If hairstylists just cut hair, why do they know about their clients' children's school problems? Why do they know about their clients' talents, trophies, and achievements? If hairstylists just cut hair, why do they get cookies, lasagna, and liquor from their clients? Does a doctor? Does a dentist? Do you take homemade bread to your accountant? Do you stop in to say hello if you are in your lawyer's neighborhood? Probably not.

The psy-cosmetologist/client relationship is unique. Two people are united over a cosmetic service appointment six to fifty times a year. In this process, touching, sharing, and communication between two human beings takes place.

A Theory of Personal Growth

Otto Rank, the noted psychiatrist, saw life as a constant series of choices. One choice is to grow, to move forward and to seek newness. The alternative is to retreat, to stagnate, and to cling to the past with its sameness and its predictability. We are constantly faced with making either growth or stagnation decisions in our lives.

Whether we are willing to risk growth or not is at least partially related to the significant, constant others in our lives. **With discouraging people, we are more likely to make stagnation decisions. And with close encouragement, support, and warmth from significant others, we are more likely to make courageous, growth decisions.**

Growth versus stagnation points are especially heightened during major changes in our lives. One such crucial time is the first day of kindergarten. Some children run eagerly into the new social setting, mingle with others, and adapt to life's next step (growth decision). Other children cling to mommy or daddy with tear-filled eyes, and need to be pulled like chewing gum from their parent's legs (stagnation decision).

A Psy-Cosmetologist's Application of Personal Growth Theory

I mention this example of kindergarten because of a touching experience I witnessed in a rural Chicago salon between Jonathan, a five-year-old tyke, and his stylist for three years, Jean. I've tried to capture their dialogue.

Jonathan: *You know what Jean? I start kindergarten tomorrow.*

Jean: *I know, Jonathan, and we're going to make you the most handsome boy there!*

Jonathan: *Can you make me look like Ron Kittle (a Chicago baseball player)?*

Jean: *Old Jean is going to make you look like a real baseball player. Are you excited about school, Jonathan?*

Jonathan: *I'm scared, a little. Mom says if you don't listen, the teacher gets mad and yells.*

Jean: *Sometimes doing new things is scary. But, honey, remember the first time you slept at your Aunt Paula's house and were scared of being away from home?*

Jonathan: *With Mickey and Tommy?*

Jean: *Yes. You were scared, but you wound up having fun, didn't you?*

Jonathan: *Yeah! We played baseball and stayed up real late!*

Jean: *Yes. See, I think kindergarten's going to be fun. And I wouldn't worry about the teacher getting mad and yelling. I'll just bet the teacher is going to love you. You know how much I love you, don't you?*

Jonathan: (giggles, puts hands over his little mouth)

Jean: *Okay, my little first baseman, go get them in school tomorrow, and see you in a couple.*

Jonathan: *See you in a couple, Jean. I'm gonna tell my teacher about you tomorrow. Bye.*

How much would that psy-cosmetology be worth to you if you had a son with kindergarten anxiety? How important was the actual haircut?

Jean and Jonathan:
Through the Passages of Life Together

Jean will probably see Jonathan before he graduates from elementary school, before his first junior high baseball game, before his first date, before he gets his high school class picture taken, before his graduation, and standing in the receiving line at Jonathan's wedding, telling his bride how cute Jonathan was the day before he started kindergarten. And, do you know that his bride will be very intersted in this information about her husband's early days from a person who was there, the psy-cosmetologist?

Following the therapeutic dialogue, I asked Jean if I could borrow a blow-dryer to fan the tears dry. I told her how touching it was for me to see how she helped a little tyke go forward and eagerly face a tough new life experience.

Apologetically, she replied, *Oh, I don't deserve that, I'm only a hairdresser!*

Do you think that Jean is *only* a hairdresser? Or is Jean the new psy-cosmetologist of the twenty-first century?

FACT 3: The cosmetologist has the power, the skills, and the tools to help the client look and feel more attractive, and in turn, more confident.

A third uniqueness about the psy-cosmetologist/client relationship is that the helper has the power and ability to impart beauty, which could also mean greater confidence.

A doctor tends to the medical health of a patient. A cosmetologist can't. A dentist tends to the dental health of a patient. A cosmetologist can't. An accountant tends to the fiscal health of a client. A cosmetologist can't. A lawyer tends to the legal health of a client. A cosmetologist can't. The psy-cosmetologist or the P.H.D.—*Professional Hair Designer*—tends to the hair, skin, and nail health of a client, which the doctor, dentist, accountant, lawyer, teacher, electrician, plumber, librarian, and chairman of the board can't. Beauty is the cosmetologist's area of expertise, his or her "niche".

A clean bill of health from a doctor can give confidence about one's internal organs and general health. A cavity-free checkup can give one confidence for six months about one's teeth and gums. Balanced, accurate books can give one confidence against an IRS audit. A roofer's skills can reassure one that the rain and the squirrels won't be living with the family. Victory in a court case can give one confidence about staying out of jail.

Keep in mind that the psy-cosmetologist gives confidence in *self*, the very core of the personality. And when you have self-confidence, you can get almost anything you want!

Artists of People

The master diamond cutter, so valued in our society, works only on a *thing*, a stone, a diamond. A cosmetologist designs a breathing, alive *human being* who shines as a result of the treatment. The client can change and can feel much more than the shiny stone.

The greatest artists in the world, the Van Goghs, the El Grecos, the Picassos, did their work on mere canvas. The cosmetologist's canvas is a *person*. The canvas of an artist does not ask to look a certain way. The canvas is discarded if too many errors are made. **The salon artist works not on mere canvas, but on a fellow human being,** who in some cases asks to look a certain way and certainly cannot be discarded, but lives on as a continual reminder of the artist's work.

The Psy-Cosmetologist's Mission:
To Help People Feel, Look and Be Beautiful

CAN YOU TELL US A GREATER MISSION THAN THIS?

Watch people when they come into a salon. Watch them when they leave. The difference, whether measured in facial expression, height of chin, extroverted attitude, or proud shoulders, was a professional hairstylist who gave time, attention, touch, caring, and a hairstyle. How important is that contact to the client's confidence?

- How many people stay home instead of going out for the evening because they feel that they don't look their best? Yet, the following night, after they visit their hairdressers, they *will* go out.
- Stylists can tell when one of their clients met someone new on the social scene by the "can you fit me in today, as soon as possible?" syndrome.
- Before the president of the United States goes on TV to make a firm statement to the world, who do you think will be one of the last people to see him before his talk?
- Many stylists say that the elderly person who goes shopping

once a week does so only on the day of his or her visit to the salon.

- One salon owner and stylist we know combs and works on the hair of a major midwestern city mayor every morning before his day at city hall. The mayor's chauffeur told one of us that this is an important part of his day, to give him the lift he needs to lead his people.

- Lew McNeil, a hairstylist from Minneapolis, Minnesota, is the only reason why a psychotically depressed patient could get out of the mental hospital every five weeks. Lew knew how to cut to avoid painful reminders of electro-shock therapy. He was told that the patient remained free from depression for several days after she returned from her haircut appointment.

We could go on and share another thousand stories to support the cosmetologist's power to help people *feel* and *be* beautiful, and how feeling beautiful gives confidence. So could you, if you just stop to think about it.

A Springfield, Illinois barber-stylist friend, Bernie K., observed, *People don't come to us for a haircut. They come to us for courage, confidence, and hope.*

Let us simply ask you this: If Susie Harris is going to be at the altar early tomorrow morning, where will she be today? With the doctor? With the engineer? With the chairman of the board? NO! She'll be with the second most important person in her life for a period of time—her hairstylist.

The psy-cosmetologist touches people, removes their masks and defenses, is with them on a regular, ongoing basis during crucial life periods, and has the tools to make people be and feel beautiful, thus confident. Whew!!

PSY-COSMETOLOGISTS AND MENTAL HEALTH RESOURCES

We like to consider ourselves as working in a field of study that we have introduced as *Psy-Cosmetology*. It is a blend of the disciplines of human behavior and cosmetological science. We feel that it will be one of the most exciting areas of study in the future of both disciplines—psychology and cosmetology.

Already it has started. One hairstylist in Vancouver, British Columbia, opened up a salon in the front of a building, and her psychologist friend established his practice in the back of the same building. She told us, *His knowledge of the mind and my knowledge of the body were a natural combination.*

Progressive mental health agencies, psychologists, social

workers, and psychiatrists are finding a viable information center in the professional cosmetology and barber-styling fields. **Cosmetologists touch people and see many people many times in a year, and are among the first members of a community to sense changes in their clientele's personalities. It is this personality change that is the key to detecting potential problems. Professionals in behavioral science need the information that cosmetologists can supply to help improve the mental health of the community.** Keep these facts in mind:

- The cosmetologist sees people who experience a series of stressful events.
- The cosmetologist sees people whose mood swings are pronounced.
- The barber-stylist sees people who show immaturities.
- The barber-stylist sees anxieties and loss of coping skills.
- The cosmetologist sees people who are potentially dangerous expressing hostilities toward others.
- The barber-stylist sees people who are losing touch with reality and live in fantasy worlds.
- The cosmetologist sees the elderly person who can barely get around and needs help. That help might be available in the community. The cosmetologist could help make the right connections.
- The barber-stylist sees the abusive parent.
- The cosmetologist sees the woman whose premenstrual tensions cause unusual behaviors.
- The barber-stylist sees the person who behaves suspiciously on the verge of destruction.
- The cosmetologist sees the pregnant mother who is smoking and drinking incessantly.
- The barber-stylist sees the little child whose doggie was hit by a car.
- The cosmetologist sees the person who is going through divorce.
- The barber-stylist sees the teenager who has lost a parent.
- The cosmetologist sees the girl who no one asked to dance at the Saturday night dance.
- The cosmetologist sees the person living in the fast lane of drug addiction.

The cosmetologist is one of the community's most likely sources to help people obtain the professional assistance they need.

George J. Vogel, the insightful director of the Council on Chemical Abuse in Berks County, Pennsylvania, put it even more bluntly:

There is no place, that's right, no place in our communities that has more of a "touching" impact on the lives of so many than in a salon. A trained hairstylist or barber can tell us more about the neighborhood, its people, its stresses, and what is going on there. This information is valuable from a preventative mental health perspective. I predict that many behavioral scientists of the future will start exploring this rich but unexplored potential mental health pulse point in the salon. Already we have started making our plans.

When a family member has a drug or alcohol problem, everyone in the family is affected. Many times, people share a confidence with their hairstylist or barber that allows their clients to talk about many of the family problems, including those caused by addiction. This being the case, a well-trained hairstylist or barber could be an invaluable resource to such a family. In fact, the hairstylist or barber could be one of the most overlooked human resources in our communities.

Imagine the countless number of tragedies and the needless suffering that could be averted through the earlier identification of such problems. If this early identification is possible, and I truly believe it is, traditional means of identifying such people in need of help could become outdated. In fact, there may be no place, that's right, no place in our communities that holds more potential for identifying people and families in need of drug or alcohol services than does the neighborhood salon.

The Cosmetologist Is Not a Psychologist

One vital point that can't be made strongly enough is this: **psy-cosmetologists are not trained to be therapists.** A therapist's training involves at least a master's degree in counseling, social work, or psychology. Many cosmetologists attempt to solve clients' problems and to be psychologists. This is an error and is beyond the scope of their training. Trained psy-cosmetologists are given rigid guidelines about what they can do to help their clients, how they can recognize potential problems, and how they can encourage clients to seek appropriate, professional assistance. But, they can never be psychologists. It is of utmost importance that professional hair designers stay within their area of expertise.

HIGHLIGHTS FROM CHAPTER 1

After observing the powerful role the professional hair designer plays in the lives of people in the community, I (Lewis Losoncy) decided to gain a better understanding of that special and unique relationship. For close to a decade, I worked with beauty and barber supply manufacturers, distributors, salon owners, managers, stylists, cleansing technicians, receptionists, specialists, and especially, salon clientele. I combined my findings with the practical expertise of cosmetologist Donald Scoleri's twenty-four years in the salon industry. Chapter 1 has discussed those findings.

Three primary reasons explain the uniqueness of the psy-cosmetologist's relationship with the client:

1. **THE PSY-COSMETOLOGIST TOUCHES THE CLIENT**. Touch is a vital human need, and very few people's touch needs are met. The most natural spot in the whole community for touch needs to be satisfied is the salon! In some cases, the stylist is the only one who touches a client in his or her adult life. Touch builds trust.

2. **PROFESSIONAL HAIR DESIGNERS SEE THEIR CLIENTS ON A REGULAR, ONGOING BASIS, AND BEFORE MOST OF THEIR IMPORTANT LIFE EVENTS.** Besides touching, which builds trust, hairstylists see their clients six to fifty times a year for sometimes more than twenty years, and are with them during family births, family deaths, and all emotionally provoking events in between. This frequency of close contact leads to a special relationship unique to the styling profession.

3. **COSMETOLOGISTS HAVE THE POWER, THE SKILLS, AND THE TOOLS TO MAKE PEOPLE BE AND FEEL BEAUTIFUL AND, IN TURN, CONFIDENT.** Along with touching to build trust and frequency of contact, professional hair designers are the top beauty experts in the lives of their clients. When you look good, you feel good, you feel confident and hopeful. Stylists give beauty on a physical level, and hope and confidence on a metaphysical level.

DOES ANY OTHER PROFESSION IN THE WORLD MAKE A GREATER CONTRIBUTION TO SOCIETY?

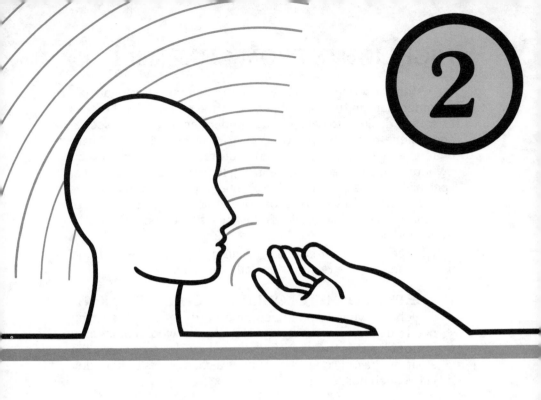

2

Qualities Of The New Psy-Cosmetologist

PROSPERITY AND RESPECT

The professional salon industry is coming of age. The proud whitecaps of a whole new wave in the cosmetology profession are being sighted in the distance. The powerful swells are dancing closer to the shoreline each and every day. The approaching wave is cresting with positive news of a future of plenty. It is already hinting that **the salon industry will have a tomorrow filled with long-deserved community respect, full professional status, financial opportunities, and growth and prosperity in new directions.** Yes, insightful future salon visionaries realize that the psy-cosmetologists of their profession are on the threshold of the biggest boom yet. The twenty-first-century hairstylist will be determined to do simply what has to be done to ride this new wave. The "house of mediocrity" will be too small for the new psy-cosmetologist to settle in.

Reaping the Benefits of Change

This revolution of the twenty-first century will not be the first major change in the industry. There were previous times of change; some presented opportunities, some presented temporary setbacks. Most notable, of course, was the precision haircutting revolution of the 1970s. Those who read the waters of that change without resistance, charted their courses accordingly, and rode the new wave of precision haircutting were the ones who reaped the benefits of its power.

Many salon artists can also remember the social revolution brought on by rock groups such as the Beatles in the 1960s. The professionals who failed to read that wave of change stubbornly sat by and waited for the past to return. As we all know now, it didn't. Other far-sighted, growth-oriented visionaries of the future saw the need for change, captured the clientele that was out there, and found ways of preparing for the blossoming of the profession.

In the past revolutions, it was simply a matter of a realistic and positive attitude toward existing conditions and the creativity to successfully take advantage of those trends in the most productive way possible. The early maturers made the necessary adjustments and put their nets down where the fish were heading, so to speak. As we all know, it's easier to catch fish where they are.

A New Vantage Point

No less significant is this new revolution, the Human Revolution of the twenty-first century. And no less significant is the role of the professionals' attitudes toward what they can already dimly see in the distance. It has already begun! This revolution, however, differs from the gyrations of the past in that **the Human Revolution is a radical transformation not in how one cuts, but rather in *who one is*.** This new wave of the twenty-first century is not a change in styling skills, but rather a change in attitude toward oneself, one's clients, one's profession, and most fundamentally, a change in one's very view of life. The professional salon industry stands proudly on the welcome mat of the Human Revolution.

The Human Revolution

The Human Revolution is making an uncompromising demand upon all professions for more "human" treatment of clients. Medical schools, for example, are now teaching doctors of the future how to be more humane, more patient-oriented. The old-time house call will be making its reentry in the twenty-first century. Dental schools are now helping young dentists learn to relate not just to the teeth of the people in their chairs, but also to the *persons* who decide to sit in their chairs. Businesses spend millions annually teaching their sales personnel how to communicate with the *person* who decides to buy from them (or decides to buy from someone else!). Industry invests no fewer dollars in helping managers to manage not systems alone, but the *people* in their systems. Encouraging managers see more productivity, more creativity, more cooperation, and better morale in their employees. School teachers are spending more and more time in school and in in-service training, not learning more about Ponce de Leon or grammar, but learning how to influence, inspire, and encourage the very person of the learner. *PEOPLE* **MAKE THE DIFFERENCE.** In most professions, the Human Revolution is here!

THE SALON INDUSTRY, THE HUMAN REVOLUTION, AND THE CONSUMER

In the professional salon industry, it is no different. The Human Revolution is demanding a new type of person who will be awarded the right to hold shears, who will have the opportunity to experience the thrill of being called a professional hairdresser, and who will have the governing board's approving nod to be part of the cresting of a profession. Cosmetology and barber-styling schools are already making plans for the development of a new breed of "humanized" students. In his 1983 keynote address at the National Association of Cosmetology Schools convention in New Orleans, Dr. Lew Losoncy stated his observations:

The Human Revolution is an idea whose time has come in the professional salon industry. The better schools, in general, are doing a relatively good job of teaching students how to cut. MODERN SALON Magazine reported that 96% of the salon clients they surveyed were satisfied with their haircuts. And we can proudly state that no less than 93% of the salon clients reported being pleased with the coloring or perming they received. You, as school owners, are to be congratulated for your contributions of the past.

The newest direction and focus for our future in this Human Revolution is on developing the person of the student who will be working with the person of the future client. Yes, while it is true that better than nine out of ten clients are pleased with their cuts, perms, coloring, and manicures, stylists lose clients because of human factors.

An eye-opening actuality is this: ***Better than two out of three clients who leave one stylist to go to another stylist do so because of the stylist's poor attitude, insensitivity, unprofessionalism, negativism, irresponsibility, or self-centered behavior.*** *Stylists receive hundreds of hours of training in technical skills and very little training, education, and experience in human relations skills and attitudes. And yet the research at SALON TODAY Magazine reveals that when a stylist is asked what consumes most of his or her time in the course of a typical day, we hear a people-related, not a hair-related, answer.*

24

Also consider the fact that **more stylists leave the profession or leave a particular salon based on people or social factors than leave because of an inability to cut, color, or perm.** Salon owners and managers want students with a service-oriented attitude, an ability to communicate, a desire to grow and be responsible, and the ability to work with others.

The schools need to find ways to prepare students who have the ability to quench the thirst of the Human Revolution. It will demand psy-cosmetologists. **Psy-cosmetology must start in the schools.** It is you as schoolmen who must plant the first seeds to the Human Revolution. It won't go away, but the Human Revolution will eagerly allow you to join and to contribute. It's an idea whose time has come.

Meeting Human Needs

Supporting the importance of the Human Revolution, the authors of *In Search of Excellence,* Thomas Peters and Robert Waterman, reported on their research into the common factors present in America's top corporations. If there were a commonality woven throughout the fabric of the biggest companies, that element could be incorporated in the future plans of our profession. Interestingly, one of the most significant commonalities discovered was totally consistent with the Human Revolution. The brilliant researchers found that **America's top businesses were obsessed with achieving a "closeness to the customers" they serve.** Peters and Waterman wrote:

In observing the excellent companies, and specifically the way they interact with customers, what we found most striking was the consistent presence of obsession. This characteristically occurred as a seemingly unjustifiable over-commitment to some form of quality, reliability and service. Being customer-oriented doesn't mean that our excellent companies are slouches when it comes to technology or cost performance. But they do seem to us more driven by the direct orientation to their customers than by technology or a desire to be a low cost producer.

The Client As Ultimate Boss

The Human Revolution touches all industries, accentuating very clearly the fact that the customer or client is in the driver's seat. The twenty-first century salon will be staffed with people who realize the vast potential in being human-oriented. True psy-cosmetologists will be fully aware of what lecturer and Vancouver salon owner Geoffrey Lane calls "the other cutting edge," the *human* side of the cutter.

Lew Young, President of the Diebold Group, spoke of unsuccessful companies' failure to be customer-oriented:

Probably the most important management fundamental that is being ignored today is staying close to the customer to satisfy his needs and anticipate his wants. In too many companies, the customer has become a bloody nuisance.

Another best-seller, *Megatrends,* authored by John Naisbitt, discussed the power that the consumer has to choose between options. Commenting on the major trends that are shaping our society of the future, Naisbitt noted that one difference between the worlds of yesterday and tomorrow is that we are living in a multiple-option world. We know we can choose how to spend our time and money. But we didn't always have these options. Naisbitt wrote:

Personal choices for Americans remained rather narrow and limited from the postwar period through much of the 1960s. Many of us lived the simple lives portrayed in such television series as "Leave It To Beaver" and "Father Knows Best." Father went to work, mother kept house and raised 2.4 children. Not anymore. In a relatively short time, the unified mass society has fractionalized into many diverse groups of people with a wide array of differing tastes and values, what advertisers call market-segmented, market-decentralized society.

Remember when bathtubs were white, telephones were black, and checks were green?

People are aware that they live in a multiple-choice society. They recognize the fact that they have choices, and they are assertive enough to use their options. The public is more educated than ever, will turn back poorly cooked steaks to the chef, will call a consumer protection agency if mistreated, and will even ask for a second doctor's opinion about their medical conditions. And, yes, the people in the public will, and are, changing hairstylists if they don't receive human treatment in the salon. In the twenty-first century, they will be even more educated and more financially sound. They will spend more than ever, but more wisely, and only in places where their human needs are met.

Giving More Than a Haircut

The twenty-first century will be a time of boom if we are ready to accept its challenge, its very dare to us to give

more than just a haircut to that person who selected us. Psy-cosmetologists see the dancing wave of the Human Revolution coming closer and are looking for ways to prepare themselves to ride the new crest. But how can one prepare? What are the characteristics necessary for the new era of styling? What will a psy-cosmetologist need in addition to excellent haircutting, perming, coloring, and manicuring skills? What psychological, human-related skills will be necessary to help one capture a lion's share of the treasures of the twenty-first century?

Characteristics of the 21st Century Psy-Cosmetologist

- **Client-Centered Professional**—being a creative hairstylist who concentrates on satisfying each client's individual needs.
- **Service Scientist**—projecting a warm, positive attitude of service to the client.
- **Asset Focuser**—focusing on the existing assets and potential in the client's hair, skin, and nails.
- **Optimistic Realist**—achieving a nice balance between being an optimist and a realist.
- **Responsible Self-Starter**—taking the responsibility and the initiative for professional development.
- **Risk Taker**—having the courage to be imperfect while moving toward one's goals.
- **Community Contributor**—reaching out to develop the potential in the community.
- **Cooperative Team Member**—participating as an involved, cooperative salon team member.

CLIENT-CENTERED PROFESSIONALS

Experts in any profession have a natural bias for recommending specific treatments and procedures that they are most aware of or do well. For example, if four people, one a nutritionist, one a psychologist, one a minister, and one an aerobics teacher, all observed the same depressed person, chances are each would arrive at a different explanation as to why the person was depressed and how to go about remedying the problem. The nutritionist would probably recommend a new diet, perhaps with less salt in it. The psychologist might recommend some form of psychotherapy or medication. The minister might tend to favor some form of spiritual guidance or prayer, and the aerobics instructor might recommend a type of activity to alleviate the depression.

Keep in mind that all four professionals are looking at the same person, but each is bringing his or her previous skills, background, knowledge, and orientation to the observation and recommending treatment based upon that particular range of experience and expertise. Obviously, the broader the range of the professional's experiences, the greater the help that can be provided. The range of possible recommendations is thus limited to the professional's experiences. And people tend to recommend, even within their own range of experiences, the things they do well, know best, and feel most comfortable with. Because, in general, recommendations emerge out of the professional's experiences, we call them *self-centered*.

Client-Centered Stylists Expand
Their Clients' Possibilities

Self-centered recommendations are quite frequent in the cosmetology and barber-styling professions. Hairstylists tend to recommend the cuts and colors that they have been complimented on most frequently in the past. In fact, if they feel inadequate at something like coloring, they tend to avoid making the recommendation, even if it might serve the client's needs best. Consequently, **many clients' appearances are not maximized because the self-centered recommendations are limited to what the stylists believe they can do well.**

Stylists aren't to be blamed for making self-centered recommendations. These occur in every profession. But, keep in mind that each time stylists learn a new cut at a hair show or in-salon education program, they accumulate added expertise, and all the clients in their chairs profit from this new, additional option. So, going back to our original example of a depressed person, we can see that a professional who would have expertise in all four areas, nutrition, psychology, ministry, and aerobics, would have a richer perspective and be better equipped to help the depressed person than would just a nutritionist.

And so it is that **the psy-cosmetologist with a knowledge of people is much better equipped to make an effective recommendation of a cut, perm, or color than someone with cutting skills alone.** The psy-cosmetologist has the skills of cutting, perming, and coloring PLUS the insight necessary to understand that unique individual in the chair at that moment. The psy-cosmetologist, however, doesn't start from his or her self-centered recommendation; the psy-cosmetologist starts with the client's needs. We call that form of recommendation *client-centered,* as opposed to self-centered. Contrast the difference between the haircutter and the psy-cosmetologist:

HAIRCUTTER (self-centered)	PSY-COSMETOLOGIST (client-centered)
Makes recommendations centered around personal knowledge and technical skills.	Makes recommendations centered around *client's needs.*
Has repetoire of few cuts.	Pictures as many different cuts as there are different clients.
Does robot-like cutting.	Believes in creativity, exploring alternatives, and encouraging new possibilities.
Cuts in mass production.	Individualizes cut, perm, and color.
Sees all clients in the same way.	Sees each client in unique, special ways.
Focuses on hair.	Focuses on each client's total self—physical, emotional, educational, social, athletic, and lifestyle.
Dominates by talking and telling.	Harmoniously listens and dreams with clients.
Gives similar cut each time on the same client.	Always looks for ways to refine the cut in accordance with the client's changing life, needs, and goals.

Of course, **no greater compliment can be paid to a client than to be touched by a stylist who has taken some time to listen, to envision the client's hair, facial features, physical features, and lifestyle, and to creatively put all of the feeling and information together in an individual recommendation solely for him or her.** The psy-cosmetologist's recommendation is client-centered and nests snugly in the plans of the Human Revolution. On this note, client-centered recommendations are reflections of the ultimate "closeness to the customer."

Creativity Eliminates Repetition and Boredom

One New York City stylist told us, *I'll never forget the Dorothy Hammill cut. It was a true indication of the principle that some hairstylists tend to recommend what they do well or what they just learned because it is popular. Everyone seemed to be wearing the cut regardless of what they looked like, what their lifestyle was, or what their body build was. So we had tall girls with big necklines who walked around with the Hammill cut looking like giraffes. Why? Because their hairstylists learned the Hammill cut, and the client was going to get it because the stylist could do it.* It was a fad. **Although psy-cosmetologists are fully aware of fads, they do not allow fads to dictate their work.** The real pros only allow the needs of the specific, unique human beings in their chairs to dictate their work.

An Illinois stylist-manager saw the excitement that the creative psy-cosmetologist can experience. Sharon G. commented, *I see more girls burn out because they make themselves do the same thing over and over and over again five days a week, fifty weeks a year. No excitement on the job. That's hard work. We are in one of the most creative professions in the world. When we explore with our clients various possibilities in the way they will proceed through life for the next five weeks, they, and we, can get turned on. It's like a fresh, new journey with each new client.*

We found something else very interesting about the twenty-first-century hairstylist. Whereas the robotic haircutter tends to hear clients make statements like, "Just give me the same thing," the psy-cosmetologist is more likely to hear clients ask, "Knowing me, what do you recommend?" What a compliment, perhaps the ultimate demonstration of confidence that a client can give!

So, the first characteristic that we see in the psy-cosmetologist is creative, client-centered hairstyling.

SERVICE SCIENTISTS

In the Human Revolution, when clients are more intelligent, more educated, more assertive, and more aware of their options than ever before, bright futures will be smiling on stylists who choose to live by the motto: "Service above all else." When studying the most successful stylists, something became obvious to us. **Whereas the top-earning stylists might not always be the best haircutters, in general they are the best "needs recognizers."** That is, they can spot needs in people almost instantly, and these service scientists proceed to fulfill those needs.

Going the Extra Mile for the Client

Michael R., an Edmonton, Alberta, hairstylist, was particularly adept at not losing first-time clients. The enthusiast told us, *When a new person walks through that door, that human is a total stranger in our home. Yes, the salon is our home. We feel comfortable there in the salon because we work there every day. We know where the shampoo area is, where the coffee machine is, and where the bathrooms are. The stranger opens the door, like opening the door to a strange family's home, and sees either a cold, lonely place where faces stare at him waiting for him to explain the reason for his intrusion, or a warm, inviting atmosphere of people who by their attitude invite him to come closer. Every stylist and receptionist in our home is trained to be sensitive to the new client's needs of acceptance and reassurance. We work hard at making our home their home.*

Sensitivity to the First Haircut

Psy-cosmetologists are also sensitive to a client's fears and anxieties. Tom L., a Reading, Pennsylvania, barber-stylist with a master's degree in counseling explained, *A child's first haircut and experience with this stranger holding scissors can be quite traumatic and anxiety arousing. You remember what your parents always told you about scissors and how you can get cut. So I try to untraumatize the event. I ask mother or father to bring him in once or twice before the actual first cut. Then, after cutting the parent's hair (while he or she smiles), I sit the child in the chair and say some kind words to him. Then I simply comb his hair a little and praise him for being a big boy. As he gets up, I compare him to his daddy, who just got his haircut.* A potentially traumatic experience avoided by a true psy-cosmetologist.

Little Things Mean a Lot

We've seen psy-cosmetologists who kept 3″ x 5″ cards on their clients' interests, activities, important events, birthdays, friends, lovers, and even dog's names. Rachel D. of La Mesa, California, and Jean R. of Boyertown, Pennsylvania, are just two of the many stylists we found who keep a scrapbook of photographs of their clients before important events like weddings, newspaper pictures, and so on. Rachel and Jean will be successful in this Human Revolution because of their "closeness to the customer."

Psy-cosmetologists are service-oriented stimulants. They get enthused about their clients' lives and dreams. Pam O., a Joliet, Illinois, perm pro is probably the cream of the crop at being a positive, service-oriented specialist. Never anything less than an enthusiastic smile and comment from Pam. She has an empathic excitement toward people and, like a magnet, attracts an ever-growing clientele. Little things, like a smile and a positive comment, mean a lot. Pam is one of the leaders in the Human Revolution.

Positive Service to the Elderly

We'd like to single out an important client group, the elderly. We've seen some very touching and sensitive experiences of service-oriented salons who make an effort to understand the psychology of aging. The issue is a crucial one, for **in the twenty-first century the largest part of the population will be over forty years of age.** With the advancement of medical science, two trends have occurred. One is that the birth control pill has led to fewer births, but advances in controlling heart disease, polio, some forms of cancer, and other diseases have kept people living longer than ever. There are fewer young people and more and more elderly people, and the aging trend will continue. **Psy-cosmetologists who desire to build and maintain clientele will work vigorously to keep their doors open to this proliferating market.** Many stylists express problems in working with the elderly, and their main complaint is centered on the attitude of impatience that the elderly person sometimes expresses.

Don't Be Fooled By What They Say

A Toms River, New Jersey, salon-owner husband-and-wife team shared with us, *The reason the elderly act like they have so much going for them in life and get frustrated when we make them wait is because the very opposite is quite often true. Unfortunately, some believe they have very little going for them, but they don't want us to know it. They want us to think of them as first-class, not second-class, citizens, and they are. So even before they say something to us, in our salon we tell them, "I know how busy you are Mr. or Mrs. _____, so we'll get to you as soon as possible." We communicate our respect for them.*

Rumors have it that the elderly flock to the string of salons owned by Mr. and Mrs. B. An example of psy-cosmetology in action.

A poem was written by an elderly patient in a London hospital that best expresses the frustrations many senior citizens experience after living a life of being active, competent, and capable, and then finding themselves one day victims of the aging process. Although it was written to a nurse, we'd like to change a few words to have it apply as a poem written to a stylist by an elderly client. (The original author of the poem remains anonymous.)

A POEM ON LONELINESS

What do you see, stylist, what do you see?
Are you thinking when you are looking at me,
A crabby old woman, not very wise,
Uncertain of habit, with faraway eyes,
Who is late for appointments and makes no reply,
When you say in a loud voice, "I do wish you'd try!"

I'll tell you who I am as I sit here so still,
As I rise at your bidding and I lift my head at your will.
I'm a small child of ten with a father and a mother,
With brothers and sisters who love one another.
A bride soon at twenty my heart gives a leap,
Remembering the vows that I promised to keep.

At twenty-five now I have young of my own,
Who need me to build a secure and happy home.
At fifty once more babies round my knee,
Again we knew children, my loved one and me.

Dark days are upon me, my husband is dead.
I look to the future, I shudder with dread,
And I think of the years and the love that I've known.

I'm an old woman now and nature is cruel,
'Tis her jest to make old age look like a fool.
This body it crumbles, grace and vigor depart,
There now is a stone where I once had a heart.

But inside this old carcass a young girl still dwells,
And now and again my bittered heart swells.
I remember the joys, I remember the pain,
I'm living and loving all over again.

And I think of the years all too few gone too fast,
And accept the stark fact that nothing will last.
So open your eyes, stylist, open and see,
Not a crabby old 9 o'clock, look closer, see me.

Keep in mind from Chapter 1 that, in some cases, the hair-stylist may be the only person who touches a senior man or woman at that point in his or her life. So important is understanding the aging client that the psy-cosmetology training program* includes a course entitled "The Psychology of Growth and Development," which teaches students how to understand and cope with the elderly.

Understanding the elderly's or the young child's needs is going to be an important part of the Human Revolution. It is the ultimate in "closeness to the customer" with service. Our research tells us that this sensitivity to the customer in the form of attitude and service is what the clients want, and will pay for.

Positive Attitude and Service with Styling

The most basic, bottom-line questions that twenty-first-century hairstylists will want answered are: (1) If a client chooses to stop going to a certain stylist, what were the possible reasons, and (2) What were the factors that led to the client's selection of his or her new stylist? By knowing the answers to these two questions, the stylist who wants to be even more successful could design an approach for facing the "paying public."

Research at People-Media, Inc. in the form of questionnaires to over 700 clients of salons and barber shops discovered the answers to these two basic questions. The results were eye opening, to say the least. **In better than two out of three responses, the client left a stylist or sought out another stylist based on the stylist's attitude and service. The quality of the haircut was mentioned in less than one out of three instances as being a factor in stylist rejection or stylist selection.**

Here are some detailed responses to our first question: "If you recently stopped going to a certain hairstylist, what was the main reason?"

My stylist was negative, talked about her boss, the other stylists in the salon, and even the customer before me. I thought to myself, "I'll bet she talks about me after I leave."

While my hairdresser was shampooing my hair, she was arguing with the manager and banging my head against the shampoo bowl.

I'm a busy woman. I can't spend my life waiting and waiting while my stylist talks to another stylist about her personal life.

*The International Training Center for Psy-Cosmetologists is headquartered at The Gallery, 345 Morgantown Road, Reading, Pennsylvania 19611. Training is also offered in many major cities throughout the year.

She never talked. She'd say, "yes" or "no" and that would be that. You know, she is supposedly my hair care expert, and she never, ever talked about my hair and how it could look its best. I honestly felt like I do when I go to my doctor, and after my blood pressure is checked, he doesn't say a thing, just writes something down.

I have to make an early appointment because of my work. You see, I go on the road. Twice, and I should have been smart enough the first time, but twice she wasn't in at 8:15 when we agreed and apologized by saying, get this, that she was up late partying. What do I care? After the second time, I actually went to the Yellow Pages of the phone book and counted the number of salons I could go to. There were 239. I took my money elsewhere.

She didn't listen. I explicitly said, "None off the side." This girl was spaced out!

His smoking bothered me. I'm asthmatic, you see, and smoke really affects me. But I hate to be pushy and tell someone, so I just went to another stylist. I did think it was funny, though, when he told me to buy a product because it was healthy for my hair, while he was blowing yellow nicotine all over the room. It seemed a little inconsistent.

I wanted a more modern hairstyle and, frankly, she couldn't do it. I asked her when she went to a haircutting program the last time, and she couldn't remember.

It seemed like I, the customer, sort of got in the way of the business.

As you study some of the responses, it becomes obvious that poor attitude and lack of customer-oriented service with the haircut are the reasons why stylists lose clients.

Our respondents on the salon client survey not only rejected stylists because of poor attitude or poor service, but they also elected to spend their money in salons where stylists provided great client-centered services with a great attitude. Some of the responses to the question, "Why did you select the stylist you currently see?" included:

Betty is a super neat, super clean person, a real pro. From the moment you walk into her salon, she offers you a cup of coffee, she looks at your hair and she tells you some thoughts about to make it even more beautiful. If I have questions, she answers them and doesn't give you the feeling that you are taking her time.

Carl's great, He's funny. Always has a few jokes to start the day off. I could be down in the dumps on a Thursday evening, but knowing I'll be seeing Carl on Friday at 10:00 just picks me up. I never leave him feeling unhappy.

My stylist cares about me as a person. When my mother died, she sent me a card with a few comments about how much she liked my mom. I still have that card.

My picture was in the paper for winning a bowling trophy. When I came into the salon, Martha had my picture cut out and scotch-taped to the mirror. She told me that she showed it to everyone and told them proudly that I was one of her customers.

My stylist really knows hair. He can talk about it for hours, and I have learned a whole lot about hair and how to take good care of it.

I feel important and respected when I am with Marco. As soon as I walk into the salon his eyes brighten up and he makes me feel like I'm his most special customer. And yet he does the same for everyone. All the clients, whether they go to Marco or another stylist, like to talk to him. I'm amazed. He knows every client's name.

Again, it is obvious. **The Human Revolution, the twenty-first century, is demanding from professionals not only an excellent haircut, but also a positive, service-oriented attitude.** The marriage of psychology to cosmetology will be fruitful and will replenish the clientele.

The psy-cosmetologist is first of all a creative, client-centered hairstylist, and next a positive, service-oriented professional.

ASSET FOCUSERS

The twenty-first century Human Revolution is having its impact on not only the cosmetology profession, but on *all* professions that we observe. Past concepts and language so deeply rooted and accepted as part of the training and vocabulary of most professions are now being viewed with suspicion. **The shift is from focusing on the negative, the liabilities, the disease to looking at the positive, the potential, and the wellness.**

Who Wants to be Just Normal?

In the field of psychology, for example, emphasis is increasingly being placed on positive mental health, or wellness. In the past, most psychologists were trained in identifying psychopathology or recognizing diseases in what were called "patients." Then with "treatment," those "sick patients" could move closer to being called, at best, "normal." Because of that training, when a psychotherapist looked at a patient, the professional tried to tune into what was *wrong*. It was called, in many cases, "the disease." The goal was "normalcy," nothing more. Who wants to be just normal?

There is a major shift taking place in the training and in the very vocabulary of behavioral scientists in the psychological profession. Led by the early ideas of the optimistic psychiatrist Alfred Adler, and later by the far-reaching humanistic psychologists Carl Rogers and Abraham Maslow, the Human Potential Movement began looking for *what's right* with people and what ceilings they could reach for in their 30,000 days of adventure called *life*. **Normal living is no longer a worthy goal in the age of fulfillment.** The sick patient has become a client with potential for self-actualization. One such form of therapy, Encouragement Counseling, sees the goal of developing people best achieved by focusing on their assets.

In *Innovative Psychotherapies,* Lew Losoncy wrote:

Encouragement Therapy is a positive and a practical approach to developing responsible, confident and courageous clients. The main hypothesis is that regardless of which approach therapists use, in the end, the main reason why people change is because they themselves are motivated to change. The primary task in therapy then is to encourage the client's own willingness and determination to change. The raw material in therapy already exists in the client's assets, strengths, resources and potentially positive life outlook; reorganization is what is needed. Reorganization is achieved through developing the client's perceptual alternatives. With fresh perceptions of self, others and reality, clients recognize the relationship among what they think, what they tell themselves, how they feel and how they act. This powerful discovery gives them a sense of internal unity, personal control, self-power and motivation for positive movement.

Encouragement Counseling is one of the many new forms of helping that views patients as *clients*, sick as *undeveloped potential*, and sets goals of, not normalcy, but a *full life*.

Wellness versus Sickness

Not only in the field of psychotherapy is this Human Revolution occurring, but also you'll find that it has even touched the very conservative field of medicine. In medicine the same positive fruits are appearing on the trees of the profession. Wholistic medicine is calling for "personal responsibility for one's medical self." Doctors are talking about the curative powers of the human body, coupled with the human mind. Wellness, not sickness, clinics are emerging throughout the more advanced nations. The scales of medicine are making dramatic shifts, influenced by the Human Revolution.

To whom would you rather go: a doctor who tells you how poorly you look, tells you all the things that are wrong with you, or a doctor who sees the assets in your body, the strengths you have to cope with disease, and helps you develop a positive wellness-keeping plan? The Human Revolution is an idea whose time has come in psychotherapy, in medicine, and even in education.

What's Right With You?

Educators of the twenty-first century will spend more and more time and energy pointing out to students what they are doing *right* as opposed to what they are doing wrong. They will be sharing with students the potential, not the liabilities, that the learners have. They will realize the principle that you motivate, encourage, and build people, not by tearing them down, but by planting dreams inside their hearts, by showing them how high they can soar. IQs will become antiquated concepts in the twenty-first century because they are too limiting and create false ceilings. Everyone has had teachers who noticed and accented with a red pencil the two *wrong* answers rather than the eighteen *right* answers. **The negative approach seems all so primitive now in the wave of the Human Revolution's positive power.**

I (Lew Losoncy) had a few interesting experiences with dentists in my early years. Although it is assumed that a dentist's responsibility is to find dental problems, the manner in which the dentist relays that message to the client is all-crucial. One dentist after another would point out my cavities, tooth problems, and concentrate only on what was wrong, not what was *right*. I felt so humiliated when dentists would give me sermons about my "bad" teeth, or ask me such embarrassing questions as, "Don't you brush your teeth?" in front of the dental assistants.

A few years later, after having "given up" on dentists, I was talking to a gentleman I had just met at a cocktail party, and he said, *You have beautiful teeth.* I said, *What?!* He said, *You have fine looking teeth.* I was totally taken back by that. Later in our conversation, I asked him what he did for a living. He said, *I am a dentist.* I immediately asked him for his business card and made an appointment for the following week. In only four visits, all of my problems were treated, and every six months I return to this positive, asset-focusing dentist. The good doctor is truly part of the twenty-first century, of the Human Revolution in dentistry.

But now to the real point of this chapter on psy-cosmetologists of the twenty-first century. If increasingly we find psychologists seeing the assets in people's mental health, physicians looking for people's physical wellness, educators tuning in to students' positive learning potentials, and dentists emphasizing patients' healthy teeth and focusing on preventative dentistry, how do the hundreds of thousands of people in the *beauty* profession need to shift *their* thinking?

Reaching for the Assets in the Client's Hair, Skin, and Nails

We have become fascinated with how much of a stylist's time is spent talking about liabilities, deficiencies, weaknesses, and diseases in the client's hair. In fact, we have come to believe that it is second nature for the hairstylist to say, "You have a problem with dandruff," or "Your hair is unusually oily," or "Your split ends are quite noticeable." It is so second nature that many stylists think nothing of it. However, when we asked hairstylists how these same sentences felt when they listened to them empathically from the client's point of view, and experienced them sometimes within ear's range of other patrons, they felt embarrassed and humiliated.

We are not addressing this touchy issue to put anyone down; that approach is never helpful. And neither of us co-authors could condemn anyone for negative focusing because we have each been caught in the same negative trap. No one is really to blame for the negative focusing. It's just the way that hairstylists, like psychologists, doctors, teachers, and dentists of the past were trained.

Cosmetology school textbooks all had one or more chapters on "diseased hair" in its various forms, but no chapters on assets in hair. So, just as the old-time psychiatrist looked for disease or "What's wrong here?," hairstylists stroked through a client's hair with antennae extended to spot the problems. And, unfortunately, like the old-time psychiatrist's limited goal of helping the person progress from a diseased to a "normal" state, the stylist's highest goal was to make the hair normal. But, *normal* is not a very exciting description for a person's hair in the beauty industry, is it?

Kathy Finds Her Asset-Focusing Stylist

The effects of these "evil eyes" in all professions, especially the cosmetology profession, were dramatically driven home to both of us one autumn Saturday afternoon as we listened to one salon client, Kathy S., tell us of her past salon experiences. The 31-year-old, blonde sales manager told us about how she had been totally turned off by the inhumane, negative treatment she received in most of her salon experiences as a child and a teenager.

Kathy explained: *Ever since I was a young child, I would go to the salon and get abused verbally by the hairdressers. I would be repeatedly told that I have "baby-fine, limp hair" that could never be permed, never be allowed to grow long, and that my hair looked like h---! It happened over and over again. How do you think it made me feel? I mean, this stuff is growing out of my head!*

Whenever I would go anywhere, I would feel so self-conscious about my "baby hair." I felt so inferior to everyone else. And strangely, my hair inferiority came from the place you'd least expect, from the professional stylist. My mother would actually have to reassure me after I got out of the salon that it wasn't as bad as they told me. So, I'd change salons and hear from someone else, "There's not much we can do with hair like yours. But, we'll do the best we can." After years of hearing what's wrong with my hair, I decided to cut my own hair. So I saved myself hundreds and hundreds of dollars, and I didn't have to be reminded about my baby hair.

Meeting Tommy, The New Psy-Cosmetologist

Then a smile broke out on her beautiful face as she went on: *When I was twenty-seven, I decided to give the salon one more* try when I heard about this positive and sensitive man named Tommy, a stylist in northern New Jersey. After arriving at the salon, I was escorted to his chair and my tension was already building. As he came over to me with a big smile on his face, I spoke first and apologetically wished him good luck with this mess on my head. He stopped me in the middle of the apology and said, "Kathy, you have such a gorgeous face and beautiful cheek bones." While running his fingers through my hair he added, "Your hair is like silk. Cutting your hair will be a breeze." He discussed all of my special features that even I was unaware of. He helped me realize all of my hair's potential.

A few appointments later, Tommy even encouraged me to let him highlight my hair. He showed me how to take care of my hair, to respect it, to be proud of it. Not only did he change my hair, but he changed my perspective. I totally trusted him. I felt like a winner in his presence because I knew that he liked and respected my hair, and me. I would not have had the guts to apply for this sales manager's job without having found Tommy. And interestingly, my job promotion located me in another city. But every five weeks I travel four hours to see Tommy.

Doesn't what Kathy, the salon client, said make sense? Are we not more attracted to people who respect us and see what is *right* with us? **In the Human Revolution, in any profession, the successful experts will be those who are not only experts in their technical areas, but also experts in understanding people. And the first principle in understanding people is knowing that people favor the positives about themselves over the negatives.**

The Reach Concept

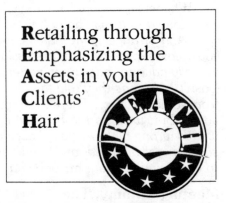

Retailing through **E**mphasizing the **A**ssets in your **C**lients' **H**air

Kathy is not alone. After several dozen interviews with salon clients, Dr. Losoncy found negative focusing to be a common experience in the discussions stylists had with their clients. As a result, in the fall of 1983, we began lecturing throughout North

America on a dramatic shift in the way cosmetologists relate with their clientele. In a major address delivered in Des Moines, Iowa, Lew Losoncy suggested:

I would like to discuss a concept barely addressed before. It appears that the cosmetology profession is sitting on the welcome mat of a brand new future in terms of the way professionals relate to their clients. The old style of relating to the disease and deficiencies of the client's hair is no longer relevant in an age when we understand how people get discouraged, leave our salons, and go elsewhere. We are on the verge, I believe, of a refreshing approach to our clients, one that builds them, builds the assets in their hair, builds our relationship with them, and even has the subconscious effect of building our very view of ourselves.

*This new way of relating to our clients literally reaches into the assets and potential in their hair, skin, nails, physical features, and lifestyles. I would like to look at that word **reach** and thus call this new way of relating to clients the REACH Concept. REACH means Relating through Emphasizing the Assets in the Client's Hair first. The REACH Concept was just a thought a few weeks ago, but has become detailed and developed and expanded by the genius yet practical mind of Donald Scoleri, who saw the power of the positive practically applied in the salon.*

Our early feedback on the concept suggests that it is being received well. Yet, the concept is such a dramataic shift from the past and is so new that it needs you, as professional cosmetologists and barber-stylists, to join in the concept's ownership by sharing your reactions to it. Keep in mind again that REACH does not naively ignore hair problems, diseases, and weaknesses. But the focus of a REACH-using stylist is, first, the positive that is present, next the potential not seen immediately, then finally the problem. But positive first, always.

A Change in Language

We believe that beauty product manufacturers of the twenty-first century will be changing their very language in the marketing of professional products. **We believe that, instead of describing products as for "oily" or "dry" hair, products will be described in terms of positive aspects and assets of hair.** We also believe that the term *home maintenance* will be a word of the past. In our surveys, clients felt the word *maintenance* carried a negative connotation like "work," "janitorial services." "house cleaning," and "sterile." We predict that more exciting phrases like "hair-care enhancements" will surface in the years to come.

We are convinced that beauty and barber-styling textbooks will be designed for psy-cosmetologists who are "asset-focused," and a chapter, at least, will be included on "recognizing beautiful hair and making it even more beautiful through your styling, coloring, or perming expertise along with your expertise in understanding the total person in your chair."

Already the REACH Client Card has been produced by the publishers of *SALON TODAY International Management Report*. The card, developed by Donald Scoleri, helps stylists look for assets and potential in clients' hair. In fact, Scoleri recommends that an "asset analysis" be done on the clients' first visit. Can you imagine your clients' reactions, especially if they are like Kathy S., when they hear what's *right* about their hair (them)?

We believe REACH is an idea whose time has come in the Human Revolution. We expect the psy-cosmetologists of the twenty-first century to be positive and optimistic people, but of course, not to the degree that they think they can fly or live unrealistically. We see the psy-cosmetologist as a professional who is quite realistic and who, indeed, has found a nice harmony between optimism and realism.

OPTIMISTIC REALISTS

What strikes us with such interest is the overall philosophy of life present in the real pros in the psy-cosmetology profession. **Across all age ranges we find stylists who are willing to see life clearly, as it is, without a need to distort, twist, bend, or shape it to fit their needs. They are realistic and thus avoid many of the frustrations of unrealistic people who live their lives based on what they think "should be" or what they "dream was" but isn't.**

This realistic acceptance of the facts, of "what really is", can be seen in many people, like the young stylists fresh out of school who know that they will be shampooing in the salon for a period of time before doing much actual styling and having their own chairs.

Sam R. of Miami, Florida, a twenty-year-old lad, explained to us, *I was thrilled to get the job here. The manager told me that shampooing will give me an excellent opportunity to meet people and to improve my ability to communicate with clients. So every* day I learn more and more about people. I'll be able to use all of these things that I am learning when I eventually get my own styling station.

Many of my friends who I went to school with started cutting hair immediately. I don't think they were ready yet. It's different than when you're on the floor in school. Some of them were put down by the clientele for being new or too young or inexperienced or for not understanding customers.

In this shampooing opportunity I have, I try to be a good listener. When they see I listen to them, it builds confidence and trust in me. When I get my station and I finally am styling, I will be more confident because of this experience. They'll see my confidence. My goal then is to be such a good listener and stylist that I will rarely lose a client.

A Realistic Salon Manager

Leona B., a recently appointed manager in a salon outside of Denver, Colorado, exemplified this same realistic handle on her job. She told us, *You know, I was appointed salon manager several months ago. Something interesting happened after I assumed the new position. All of a sudden I seemed to lose all of my friends, the other stylists who I worked with before. Like I wasn't invited out for Thursday night drinks anymore after work. Little things happened like hearing conversations stop when I entered the room.*

It upset me at first, and then I decided that not talking about my feelings wouldn't solve the problem. So I chose to face the problem quite realistically and let them know that I miss our former contacts, but I could understand if they felt differently towards me now, being a manager. I shared with each of them that realistically my job responsibilities had changed, but hopefully in other ways I hadn't. I told them that I saw the manager's job as helping the salon and the people in it to grow, and that I wanted to do just that. I wanted to help make life easier and more productive for them. I told them that my door was always open to hearing the things that were on their minds, and that if we worked together as a team, we could all enjoy our work.

Both Leona and Sam are realists. Sam knew that he needed more experience and Leona knew that she would be viewed differently because of her promotion. So, as realists do, they faced the situation "as it was."

Living Realistically

We had met some stylists who frustrated themselves with some unrealistic views about salon finances. And then we met

Sandra D., whose realistic view of management was way beyond her years. She explained, *I thought of owning my own salon, but first I realized that it would cost thousands of dollars up front. I would have all of the business headaches like managing stylists, dealing with client/stylist problems, trying to earn a profit for the business, and paying rent, supplies, heat, insurance, mainte-nance, advertising, phone, and all of the other costs.*

I looked at it very closely with my father's accountant and concluded that, bottom line, I was much better off at this time to go home at night free of worries. Besides that, the money I had saved I could put into Certificates of Deposit and collect interest rather than putting it into a business that I wasn't sure would or would not make it.

Understand, I came to that conclusion based on knowing my realistic self. I don't like 15-hour days to get ahead. I enjoy my free time, and so working for someone else is fine for me. Someone else, and I respect them, might have a personality that enjoys the work and is willing to invest their own time and money. They obviously deserve more.

Realistic cosmetologists see both sides of the story. They don't believe they are going to become millionaires just by showing up, but that a good living has to be earned. **Because of their realistic perspectives, they are less frustrated and more well-adjusted.**

Interestingly, **many of the most well-adjusted realists were also optimists.** They seemed to find a nice balance in their lives between what was realistic and what was possible for them.

Salon Optimists

Without fail, the happiest, most fulfilled, and most productive stylists were optimists. We define optimists as positive people who, very simply put, approached each day with the conviction that the problems they faced in their personal and professional lives had some sort of best solution. And with their optimism came the realistic belief that it was their job to find the answer to the problem.

Optimists Find a Way

We frequently observed in the same audience two stylists from the same salon who tackled an imaginary salon problem from two different levels of attitude, optimism and pessimism. The pessimists would give up and hopelessly throw their arms in the air. The optimists would wrinkle their foreheads in thought and stubbornly plow through the problem, because they believed that there was an answer. Then, the optimists would jot down a list of alternatives, cross out a few possibilities and add others, piggyback old ideas into newer, better ones, and soon, voila!, a solution appeared.

Whether the problem was developing a plan to increase the salon clientele, figuring out better ways to make professional recommendations, or constructing a strategy to keep every client they had, optimists always did better than pessimists. The pessimists believed that things couldn't get any better; the optimists believed things could. Both were right!

Optimistic twenty-first century hairstylists are worth their weight in gold. Not only are they the most productive, but they exhibit the most positive influence on those around them.

Lovers of Life and People

When we had the opportunity to interview some of these precious gems of attitude, we wanted to find out how they kept themselves going, with the rigors and demands of their daily salon lives. What were their daily lives like? **In all cases, the optimists were lovers and appreciators of life and its possibilities. They also loved people. They cared about and were inspired by their clientele. They craved new experiences and, somehow or other, each time they were with a long-time client they still saw him or her from a fresh perspective.**

We were totally surprised, almost dumbstruck, to find that most of these optimists did not tend to associate only with other salon personnel off the job. They had friends from all professions and all walks of life. As we thought about that finding, we realized that maybe this rich social mixture was what helped give them a fresh, nourishing perspective on people. Maybe when we work with the same people that we socialize with, we just experience a rehashing of the same old grinding problems in our after work life. This stagnation could block optimism.

The optimists tended to read more and selected their readings more carefully. They clearly weren't into scandal sheets. As one Virginia stylist said, *How can reading about the love life and divorce of a soap opera star enrich my life to the same degree as a good book or poem can?* They tended to like positive yet realistic books about life. **They tended to dress more colorfully and would experiment with new clothing and new hairstyles.** One particular manager-stylist from

Boyertown, Pennsylvania, was most exciting to visit. One week she would dress like a cowgirl, the next week like a dancer.

Optimists See What's Right

Newness was all part of the optimists' way of being. Even in restaurants, we noticed that they would try new foods while the others would go back to the hamburger. They projected an air of excitement in the way they walked, and even their vocabularies were filled with words like "great," "super," "terrific," and "no problem." They were life-givers to others, were sought out by friends as well as clients. They loved nature, and in fact, we felt that they could see things in nature that others didn't notice. One optimistic Connecticut stylist sifted through some autumn leaves, telling us about the beautiful colors. We began to see something we had previously missed. She stopped to smell the roses.

In general, these optimistic psy-cosmetologists felt comfortable with life, pleased with who they were, and that they belonged in the world. They didn't have emotional needs, interestingly enough, to make other people be different. They accepted others as they were.

When you combine the ingredients of realism with optimism in a nice balance, you find a human being with fewer frustrations, love of life, love of people, and love of self. These people are at peace. If a change needs to be made to bring their lives to a higher, more fulfilling level, they don't need to be told by someone else. Their hearts give the signal. They are self-starters. They are the new psy-cosmetologists.

RESPONSIBLE SELF-STARTERS

All of the lecturers in the professional salon industry know the self-starters, because like magic they appear almost unfailingly at all educational events. They sit in the front row with their cassette recorders and at least half a dozen new cassettes. They arrive early. They take notes like students ready to take doctoral comprehensive exams. They raise questions to find answers to take back home. They learn from their peers at break time. They, in turn, contribute their knowledge back to their profession. They are forward-stepping people who project freshness and curiosity. They introduce themselves to the lecturers with a handshake or a hug. They are truly at the head of the class and "on the move." Why not? These psy-cosmetologists are going places! They are reaching out to grasp for more of the treasures of life.

Respect for Clients

In one salon after another we see them. They don't need to be told to be on time for staff meetings or to be there by the time the first client comes to the salon. To them, time is important. Jim S., a lanky Detroit, Michigan, stylist explained to one of us his theory of time. Jim laughed, *I saw it happen once in our old downtown salon. The receptionist yelled back, "Jane, your 8:30 is here." Soon she shouted, "Jane, your 8:30 and 9:00 are both here." Still no answer. Jane wasn't there!.*

*Jane finally came in at ten minutes after 9:00, and was actually angry that, when she walked in, three clients were waiting for her! I could never understand how you can be late for a customer who is paying your way. I mean, that's not disrespect for time, it's disrespect for **people.***

The stylist went on, *I met a stylist who lived fifteen minutes by car from the salon and would leave her home five minutes before her first appointment. What was she looking for, some sort of magic? You just can't build up a good clientele if you are irresponsible.* You could *always* count on Jim S. He was a responsible self-starter.

"I'll Go to the Show"

We witnessed another of the many self-starters while consulting as salon advisors at a staffing. The manager, in following her evening agenda, turned to her staff of nine stylists and informed them of a supplier's program on haircutting being held in four weeks. Excited, she explained, *This program shows how to give a new cut based on facial features. I'd love it if maybe one or two of you could attend and perhaps bring back these new ideas of cutting to share with the others here.*

The manager looked around the room, and all but one head dropped to look at their notepads. There was a long moment of silence in the room that was only broken by the words of the youngest stylist present, appropriately named Joy. The bright-eyed girl, decked out in a green dress and red sweater, waved her hand almost apologetically and pleaded, *Well, Mrs. T., I know that I am the newest member here and that everyone else should have the right to go to the show first. But if the others are busy, I'd really like to go to the show.* She looked around as the other heads rose. She was quickly supported by one of her peers who asserted, *Yes, I think it would be great for Joy to have the experience.* Joy thanked her.

The evening ended after we conducted our program on how to work together as a team. But later, we talked about that special Joy who touched our hearts by her self-starting style and her craving for learning.

"I'm the Manager Now"

A number of years later, I (Lewis Losoncy) was lecturing in Baltimore, Maryland, and at break time a bubbling young lady came up to speak to me. She proclaimed, *I know you don't remember me, but a few years ago you were giving a workshop in our salon and we met. My name is . . .*

No need to go on, I enthusiastically interrupted. *You are Joy. Donald and I will never, ever forget your love for education. Today, your presence here proves it again. By the way, how is everyone at the salon?*

Oh, they're all doing fine, although I don't get to see them as often as I would like. You see, Dr. Lew, I'm a manager now in another salon, and between that, reading, these management seminars, and my boyfriend, I'm pretty busy.

Joy, I exclaimed, *you've made my day! Let's do someone else a big favor and make his day.* I called my partner Donald in Los Angeles and handed the phone over to Joy after he answered. He thanked me. It really did make his day.

Inspiring people like Joy can be found everywhere. You'll see them in Moberly, Missouri; Minot, Minnesota; San Diego, California; Dodge City, Kansas; Arlington, Virginia; Nashville, Tennessee; Dallas, Texas; Pocatello, Idaho; Vancouver, B.C.; Des Moines, Iowa; Columbus, Ohio; Gaylord, Michigan; Hartford, Connecticut; New Orleans, Louisiana; Decorah, Iowa; Lincoln, Nebraska; Denver, Colorado; Wheeling, West Virginia, just simply everywhere!

The professionals who are the shining stars are the responsible self-starters in every city, every salon. And there will be even more of them in the twenty-first century. And they will be even more oriented to growth and achievement of their goals than we have ever seen before in the whole industry. They will be willing to try new things rather than live in fear of making mistakes.

RISK TAKERS

In many ways, the most successful stylists we observed seemed to possess what can best be described as the spirit of a young child. Why do we say that? Well, we can't help but think that young children at birth are designed to eagerly explore their worlds. The young tyke seems to be instilled with a Columbus-type spirit for new worlds, a forward-moving, courageous drive to master the previously unmastered aspects of life through trial and error.

Encouraged by others who are not perfectionists, but who understand that it's natural to fail in trying new ideas in the school of life, the child gradually expands his or her skills. When young children fall, they simply pick themselves up and move on. They fall again, they lift themselves up again. No trauma of failure at all. Only a conviction that a mistake was made and simply needs to be corrected.

What Went Wrong with a Miracle?

When en-couraged, the child remains *courageous*. However, that original courage is more frequently lost than not. Yes, you can see a young child at age four gladly and courageously show a drawing of a horse to a friendly gathered crowd. How many adults do you know who would have the courage to draw a horse on the spur of the moment and show a group of people? **Most adults have been wounded, *dis*-couraged, and the symptoms are perfectionism, fear of the new, and low or no goals. No goals equals no future.**

Even in kindergarten we can see young children's courage in their willingness to try by raising their hands to answer questions. They could be wrong *this* time, but it doesn't make them feel personally worthless. And they can try again. But, by senior high school, you have to look in many classrooms before you see a classroom full of courageous "tryers." The hands have gone down. The original promises of life were not fulfilled for many.

What went wrong with that original miracle, the human beings who were designed for success? We believe that, for the most part, discouraging life experiences invited them to hide from challenges, to become ego-directed, to live life in defense and not in creation, and to falsely conclude that, if you make mistakes, you're worthless. We call it *being stuck in a rut, burnout, robot living,* and *depression.* It's loss of will, loss of purpose, and a constricting drive for sameness, routine.

Somehow or other this discouragement didn't happen to our sample of twenty-first-century psy-cosmetologists. As we have said before, such people have retained much of the courage of their youth and an attitude that Sophie Lazarsfeld called "the courage to be imperfect." This attitude may well indeed be the most important characteristic present in nondefensive, fulfilled living.

Ego-Centered versus Goal-Centered Stylists

One big Washington state salon made a major change in the color line they were using. The change forced the stylists to learn a whole new system of calculation totally foreign to them. Fear arose in the salon, naturally, and the stylists' anxieties over making mistakes were heightened. Gerard, a stylist in his late thirties, broke the other stylists' resistance by his courageous thoughts. *Look, I know it's going to be rough at first. It's a whole new process. It'll be hard for you and hard for me. But wasn't learning the first system hard before we mastered it? We could have given up before and we didn't. Let's plug onward and give it a try. In a matter of a brief period of time, we'll master the new system and then we'll have knowledge of both.* Gerard helped his fellow stylists take a courageous step toward mastering more of their salon world.

What is the difference between being an ego-centered person and a goal-centered professional like Gerard? From what we have seen, the differences appear to be as follows:

EGO-CENTERED STYLISTS	GOAL-CENTERED STYLISTS
Fears making mistakes, looking bad, so fears trying something new.	Loves the challenge of mastering new things.

Gives up after making a mistake or doesn't ever try because of anticipating and predicting a mistake.	Views mistakes as a very natural part of moving toward mastering new things.
Believes "Unless I'm perfect, I'm worthless." So I'll only do what I can do perfectly.	Believes "I have the courage to be imperfect and will take risks. When I make a mistake, I will simply correct it and learn from it."
Thinks when criticized by a client or a manager, "You're not so hot yourself" or goes into a shell.	Thinks when criticized, "Because I'm not perfect, maybe there is something I can learn by the criticism, and improve myself."
Resists new ideas and wants everything to remain the same.	Loves new experiences. Loves to improve and move toward mastery.
Wanders aimlessly throughout the day with no goals or very low goals.	Has specific, worthwhile goals to achieve each day.

Salons in the twenty-first century will look different because the stylists in the salons will be different. They will be goal-directed and have more of the "courage to be imperfect" in their movements toward those goals. They will see their potential by not living tied to the fear of mistakes. They will also see the potential they have not just in the salon, but also in the total community.

COMMUNITY CONTRIBUTORS

One dramatic change from the haircutters of the past to the psy-cosmetologists of the Human Revolution is their involvement and high exposure in their communities. Their newer, more accurate professional self-images signal to them that they touch many lives in the community, they have a pulse on what's going on, and they have much to contribute back to their communities. They are joining hands with doctors, lawyers, educators, and other professionals to serve on school and social service agency boards, to help establish community policies, to chaperone school class trips, and to write letters to the editors of local newspapers. Only rarely in the 1950s and 1960s would you see an occasional barber on a school board.

We have seen many psy-cosmetologists doing local radio or TV programs or writing articles for newspapers on hair or skin care. **The real pros recognize the fact that they are the hair care experts, and they want to give, they want to share their expertise with their fellow citizens.**

John and Joanne Z., owners of a Reading, Pennsylvania, salon, regularly conduct make-up classes for students in the local school district. We discovered these classes are common practice as we looked around North America. Betty E., a midwestern stylist, conducts classes for her clients on "how to parent." We've seen salons conducting aerobics, diet, cooking, even speed-reading classes for the people in their communities. **Yes, the twenty-first-century professional is aware that he or she has something to contribute and is responsible enough to make things happen.**

Stylist Teaches
Dr. Lew About Optimism

The prime example of a true twenty-first-century stylist was Peggy E. of Battle Creek, Iowa. After attending a business management lecture I (Lew Losoncy) presented in Des Moines, Iowa, Peggy asked me if I would consider coming to Battle Creek to talk to community members on the power of being optimistic.

*Dr. Lew, you just **must** come to our town of Battle Creek to talk on positive attitudes the next time you are in the area.*

Love to, Peggy. About how big is your town of Battle Creek?

Oh, we have over 800 people now, the attractive, enthusiastic salon owner proudly stated.

Well, Peggy, I cautiously replied, *with 800 people, don't get your expectations up too high. Let's shoot for maybe a dozen people or so to be at our talk.*

Oh, no, Dr. Lew! We'll have a lot more than that. A hairstylist touches a lot of lives of people who touch a lot of lives of other people.

The talk was arranged, and four months later Peggy, one of her stylists, and I drove from Des Moines to Battle Creek. By this time, Peggy had quite a full schedule prepared for me. She pulled out a slip of paper and reviewed my itinerary: *At 9:00 we have a radio program. At 10:00 you'll be with the newspaper. At 1:00 you'll be with all of the high school students of Battle Creek, at 2:30 with all of the schoolteachers, and at 7:30 you'll speak in the high school gym to the people of Battle Creek.* Peggy's goal was to raise money from admission fees to help get a new ambulance for the community. The day went really well. The people of Battle Creek, from student to bank teller, to radio disc jockey, to restaurant waitress, were all gracious.

The Power of One Psy-Cosmetologist

Finally, the evening arrived. As I prepared my notes for the lecture in the coach's office, no less than the school superintendent came to the door and said, *Peggy is ready for you.* As I walked out on the gym floor expecting twenty or twenty-five people, I saw every seat in the bleachers filled and the sides of the room loaded with additional seats to accommodate the overflow. I looked on to the gym floor, and holding a microphone to introduce me was the stylist-owner of Nu Fashion Salon of Battle Creek.

Peggy made her public speaking debut by introducing me to over 400 of her fellow citizens. Peggy made her contribution to the community. She reached out to others. Through the efforts of a hairstylist, hundreds of lives were touched, the ambulance came closer to being a reality, and the people of a town took one giant step in their respect for the power of a psy-cosmetologist! Peggy is a true twenty-first-century professional who wants to reach out into the potential in the community and become part of the growth of her society.

A Solid Citizen

There are Peggys everywhere you look. **They are people who no longer apologize for their selected profession and are proud of making their communities beautiful.** They are proud of grooming that child for his or her first day of school. They are proud of offering their salons for children on their way home from school on rainy days. They are proud of being able to squeeze a last-minute appointment in because of an unexpected romance that is potentially developing on a given day. **They are part of the Human Revolution occurring in society, and they face it not alone, they face it together. They are team players who value and respect each other in the salon and in their communities.**

COOPERATIVE TEAM MEMBERS

Clearly, salons are getting bigger than ever. **The successful stylist is a person who can work with others, one who can show respect for others and desires to help other team members grow.** This area is so important that we felt a complete chapter was needed to talk about all of the possibilities of tapping the potential of the team. So, our next chapter is all on the importance of being a salon team player and what this means to the client.

HIGHLIGHTS FROM CHAPTER 2

The Human Revolution is an idea whose time has come in all professions. Psychologists are studying positive mental health, not disease; physicians are talking about wellness, and less about sickness; schoolteachers are seeing what's right with students, not what's wrong. And in the professional salon industry, the focus is on the *person* and his or her positive assets, not on 9 o'clocks or split ends. This Human Revolution occurred because the public is more educated than ever, more assertive than ever, more aware that they have options to go wherever they choose to spend their money.

Research demonstrates that, although people (better than 90 percent) are pleased with their cuts, color, or perms, they leave a particular salon or stylist because of human factors like negative attitude, poor communication, or irresponsibility. Peters and Waterman, authors of *In Search of Excellence,* found that one of the biggest factors leading to the success of America's top corporations was "closeness to the customer." All factors in society point to the same conclusion: **the salons and stylists who will be most successful in the twenty-first century will be those who understand people as well as styling.** They will be psy-cosmetologists. Their education will increasingly provide a balance between the understanding of human behavior and the technical skills of styling.

Successful twenty-first-century psy-cosmetologists will be professionals who are moving toward (1) being creative, "client-centered" stylists; (2) taking a positive, service-oriented approach toward clients; (3) focusing on the assets and potential in the client's hair, skin, and nails; (4) achieving a nice balance between being optimists and being realists; (5) being responsible self-starters who crave education; (6) having the "courage to be imperfect" in moving toward goals; (7) reaching out into the potential in the community; and (8) participating as involved, contributing salon team members.

In Chapter 1 we explored the intensity and uniqueness of the stylist/client relationship: A stylist has a license to touch people, and does so six to fifty times a year for a period of years. In this chapter we highlighted the fact that people in the cosmetology profession who see a wider vision of their talents are increasingly incorporating knowledge from the field of psychology to better or more fully service their clientele. These are the new psy-cosmetologists. How can you benefit from this experience called psy-cosmetology? Psy-cosmetology is a revolutionary break-through in self-modification.

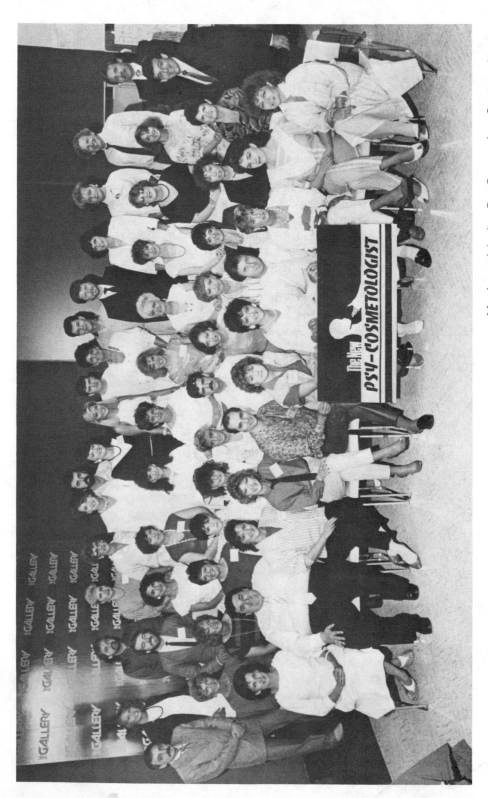

Members of the first Psy-Cosmetology Seminar class,
held at The Gallery, Reading, Pennsylvania, June 9 - 11, 1985.

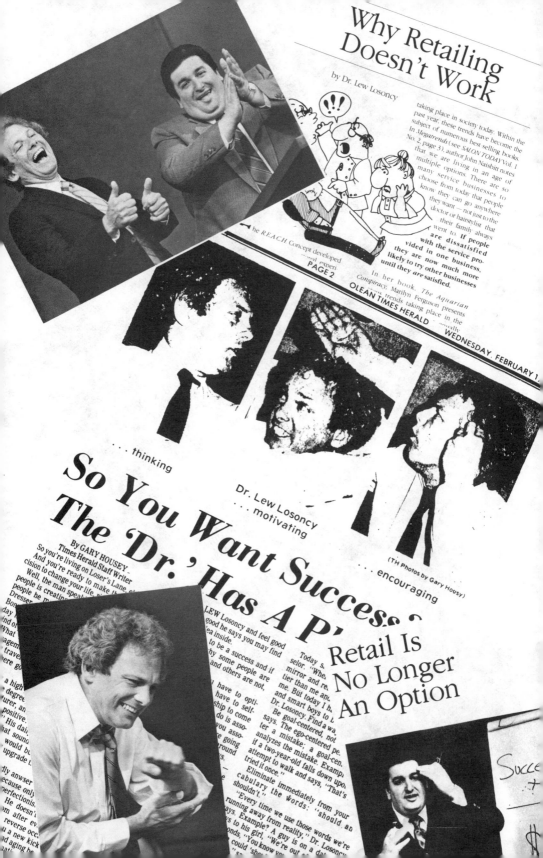

Why Retailing Doesn't Work

by Dr. Lew Losoncy

taking place in society today. Within the past year, these trends have become the subject of numerous best selling books. In *Megatrends* (see *SALON TODAY* Vol. 1, No. 2, page 3), author John Naisbitt notes that we are living in an age of multiple options. There are so many service businesses to choose from today that people know they can go anywhere they want — not just to the doctor or hairstylist that their family always went to. **If people are dissatisfied with the service provided in one business, they are now much more likely to try other businesses until they *are* satisfied.**

In her book, *The Aquarian Conspiracy*, Marilyn Ferguson presents ... some trends taking place in the ...

the REACH Concept developed
...ual experi...
PAGE 2

OLEAN TIMES HERALD WEDNESDAY, FEBRUARY 1.

... thinking

Dr. Lew Losoncy
... motivating

... encouraging

(TH Photos by Gary Housy)

So You Want Success
The 'Dr.' Has A P'...

By GARY HOUSEY
Times Herald Staff Writer

So you're living on Loser's Lane, ... And you're ready to make the ... cision to change your life. ...

Well, the man speak... people be...

Bon...
day ...
and o...
What ...
agem...
trave...
here go...

a high ...
degree, an...
turer, an...
positive. ...
His dai...
hat soun...
would bu...
upgrade L...

tly anwser ...
ecause only ...
erfectionis...
He doesn'...
om after ev...
reverse occ...
a new kick ...
ad aging ...
at!...

LEW Losoncy and feel good
good he says you may find
ea inside
hy some people are
and others are not,

have to opti-
have to self-
ship to come
do is asso-
you going
... round ...
s.

Today s...
selor. "Whe...
mirror and re...
tier than me an...
me. But today I h...
and smart boys to b...
Dr. Losoncy. Find a wa...
Be goal-centered, not...
says. The ego-centered pe...
analyzes the mistake. Examp...
attempt to walk and says, "That's ...
if a two-year-old falls down upon ...
tried it once."

Eliminate immediately from your
cabulary the words: "should an...
shouldn't."

"Every time we use those words we're
running away from reality," Dr. Losoncy
says. Example? A guy is on a da...
ays to his girl, "We're out ...
onds, "You know yo...
could 'sho...

Retail Is
No Longer
An Option

Succe...
+
...

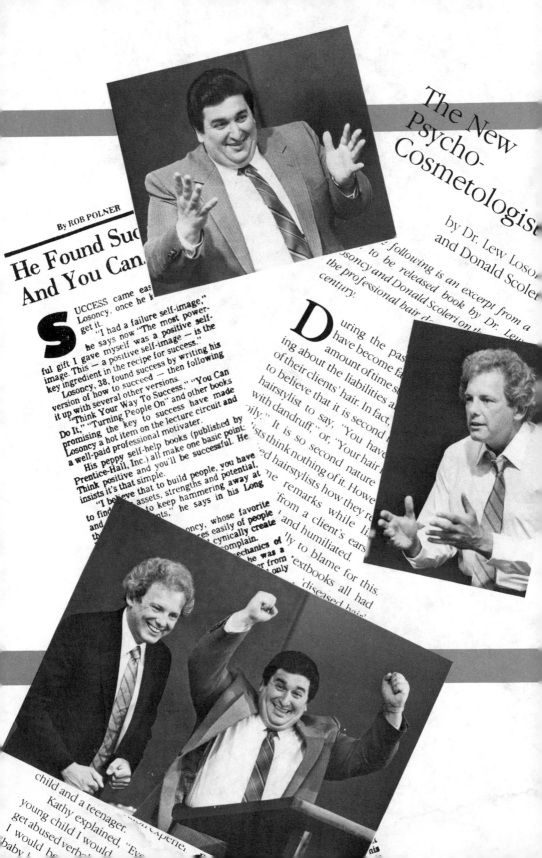

The New
Psycho-
Cosmetologist

by Dr. Lew Loson...
and Donald Scoler...

...e following is an excerpt from a
...to be released book by Dr. Lew
...soncy and Donald Scoler ion th...
the professional hair d...
century.

By ROB POLNER

He Found Suc...
And You Can...

SUCCESS came eas...
Losoncy. once he k...
get it.
"I had a failure self-image,"
he says now "The most power-
ful gift I gave myself was a positive self-
image. This — a positive self-image — is the
key ingredient in the recipe for success."
Losoncy, 38, found success by writing his
version of how to succeed — then following
it up with several other versions.
"Think Your Way To Success," "You Can
Do It," "Turning People On" and other books
promising the key to success have made
Losoncy a hot item on the lecture circuit and
a well-paid professional motivater.
His peppy self-help books (published by
Prentice-Hall, Inc.) all make one basic point:
Think positive and you'll be successful. He
insists it's that simple.
"I believe that to build people, you have
to find ... assets, strengths and potential,
and ... to keep hammering away at
th... ...nts," he says in his Long

...oncy, whose favorite
...es easily of people
...cynically create
...complain.
...echanics of
...he was a
...r from
...only

During the pas...
have become fa...
amount of time s...
ing about the liabilities a...
of their clients' hair. In fact,
to believe that it is second...
hairstylist to say, "You hav...
with dandruff," or, "Your hair...
oily." It is so second nature...
...ists think nothing of it. Howe...
...ed hairstylists how they r...
...ne remarks while li...
...from a client's ears...
...and humiliated...
...ly to blame for this...
...extbooks all had...
...diseased hair...

child and a teenager.
Kathy explained, "Ev...
young child I would...
get abused verb...
I would be...
baby...

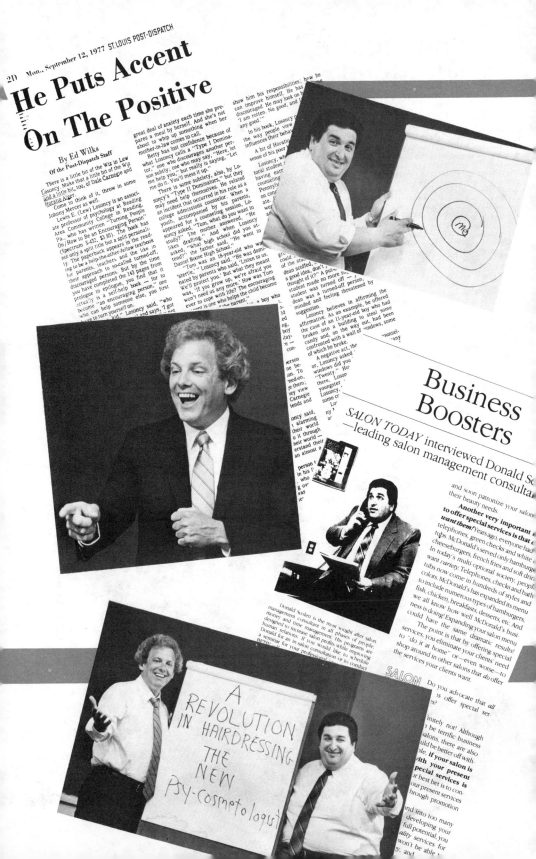

He Puts Accent On The Positive

By Ed Wilks
Of the Post-Dispatch Staff

There is a little bit of the Wiz in Lew Losoncy. Make that a little bit of the Wiz and a little bit, too, of Dale Carnegie and Horatio Alger.

Come to think of it, throw in some Johnny Mercer as well.

Lewis E. (Lew) Losoncy is an associate professor of psychology at Reading Area Community College in Reading, Pa., who has written "Turning People On/How to Be an Encouraging Person" (Spectrum S-432, $3.95). The book has not only a split title but a split personality. The paperback appears in the reading to be a help-the-other-fellow textbook for parents, teachers and the like in their approach to so-called turned-off, discouraged persons. But by the time you have completed the 143 pages from prologue to epilogue, you find that it actually is a self-help book — for to become "an encouraging person," one who can help someone else, you first have to turn yourself on.

... kid," Losoncy said, "I got ... and says, 'I got ... not ...

great deal of anxiety each time she prepares a meal by herself. And she's not about to whip up something when her mother-in-law comes to call.

Betty has lost confidence because of what Losoncy calls a "Type I Dominator," one who discourages another person subtly; one who may say, "Here, let me help you," but really is saying, "Let me do it. You'll mess it up."

There is some subtlety, also, by Losoncy's "Type II Dominators," but they may need help themselves. He related an incident that occurred in his role as a college admissions counselor. When a youth, accompanied by his parents, appeared for a counseling session, Losoncy asked, "Tom, what do you want to study?" The mother answered, "He likes drafting." And when Losoncy asked, "What high school did you attend?" the father said, "He went to Daniel Boone High School."

"Tom was an 18-year-old who was 'sterile,'" Losoncy said. "He was dominated by parents who said, 'Listen to us. We'll protect you. But what they meant was, 'If you grow up, we're afraid you won't need us any more.' How was Tom ever to cope with life? The encouraging ... is one who helps the child become ... the parent."

show him his responsibilities; how he can improve himself. He has ... discouraged himself. He may look on himself and say, 'I am rotten. No good, and ... any good.'"

In his book, Losoncy ... the way people view ... influences their behavior ...

A bit of Horatio ... sense of his poor ...

Losoncy, who ... toral student ... having, earned ... counseling ... Pennsylva ... on con ... ate ...

... could ... dean scoffed, "I ... a good idea, don't ... thought of it?" A put- ... student made no more sen ... dean was a turned-off person, ... minded and feeling threatened by suggestion.

Losoncy believes in affirming the affirmative. As an example, he offered the case of an 11-year-old boy who had broken into a building to steal some candy and, on the way out, had been confronted with a wall of windows, some of which he broke.

A negative act, thr ... or, Losoncy asked ... windows did you ... "Twenty." Ho ... there," Loson ... youngster ... Losoncy ... some co ... Lo ... ny ... a ...

Business Boosters

... and soon patronize your salon ... their beauty needs.

Another very important ... to offer special services is that c ... want them. Years ago, everyone had ... telephones, green checks and white ... tubs. McDonald's served only hamburge ... cheeseburgers, french fries and soft drin ... In today's multi-optional society, peopl ... want variety: Telephones, checks and bath ... tubs now come in hundreds of styles and ... colors. McDonald's has expanded its menu ... to include numerous types of hamburgers, ... fish, chicken, breakfasts, desserts, etc. And ... we all know how well McDonald's busi ... ness is doing! Expanding your salon menu ... could have the same dramatic results!

The point is that by offering special ... services, you eliminate your clients' need ... to 'do it at home' or—even worse—to ... shop around in other salons that do offer ... the services your clients want.

SALON   Do you advocate that all ... s offer special ser- ...

... initely not! Although ... be terrific business ... salons, there are also ... ... ble, if your salon is ... with your present ... special services is ... r best bet is to con- ... our present services ... hrough promotion ... ... nd into too many ... developing your ... full potential, you ... ality services for ... won't be able to ... and ...

Donald Scoleri is the most sought after salon management consultant in all phases of people, money and time management. His programs are designed to increase salon profits while improving human relations. If you would like to schedule Donald for an in salon consultation or to conduct a seminar for your profession ...

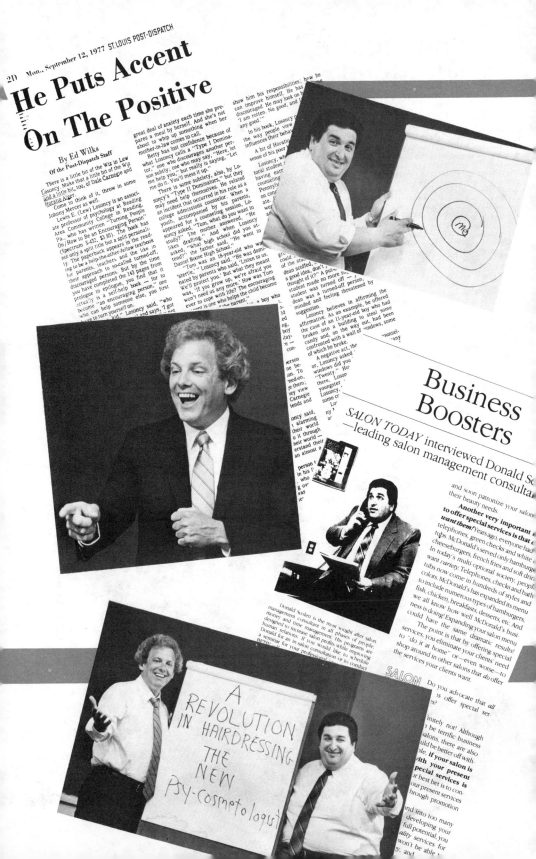

A REVOLUTION IN HAIRDRESSING THE NEW Psy-cosmetologist

You Can Be A Motivating Leader

by Dr. Lew Losoncy

Is good leadership an innate talent or a learned skill? *SALON TODAY* sought the expert opinion of Dr. Lew Losoncy, author of *You Can Be The Motivating Leader*, to be published by Prentice-Hall in early 1985 . . .

It was said that Walt Disney could wring out the creativity from his artists' minds long after they themselves thought that their ideas had dried up. One could say that he helped people go a step beyond to make Fantasyland a real place on a map. John Kennedy had the ability to motivate a nation of people to ask what they could do for their land. Mother Theresa inspired the world by giving nourishment to the hearts of its people. Martin Luther King, Jr., added new dimensions to the complexion of how a society looks at itself.

These leaders and many others had something in common. **They had the ability to move people to greater achievements, to appeal to the highest motives in people and to help everyone feel like an involved, contributing team member.** And their leadership techniques are relevant to anyone who is in a role where their own success depends on their ability to influence others to action.

Whether you call yourself a leader, a manager, a coach, a parent, an administrator, a president, or even if you feel like a shepherd with a flock, **your most important resource is your people. And the most crucial determinant to reaching your goals is your ability to influence, inspire, motivate and encourage your human resources.**

Those who have the talent to call others to committed action are often referred to as 'born leaders.' But they weren't born leaders the day they entered the world. No, they were born leaders the day they developed the skills to get 'in tune' with their people, the techniques to turn on the unmotivated, the knowledge to inspire the irresponsible.

the p...
salon...
ground...
job train...
budgeti...
schedulin...
new challe...

It was...
manager na...
her job start...
Because she...
and assertiven...., une salon
personnel start...ead all over her like an un-welcome mat.

The stress that her lack...skills caused was transformed...logical symptoms. — Inson...attacks and frequent heada...much a part of her life as h...period of only four month...successful cosmetologist le...management position, h...profession.

This sad story co...rewritten if this manage...
1. A take-charge atti...people to gain their...respect.
2. A strategy to mi...

Lewis E. Losoncy, Ed.D., is an international lecturer and consultant on encouragement, motivation and communication. Now you can learn to be a more encouraging person with Dr. Lew...video tape, *The Theo...Of Encouragement* S...order form for descr...tion and ordering inf...mation.

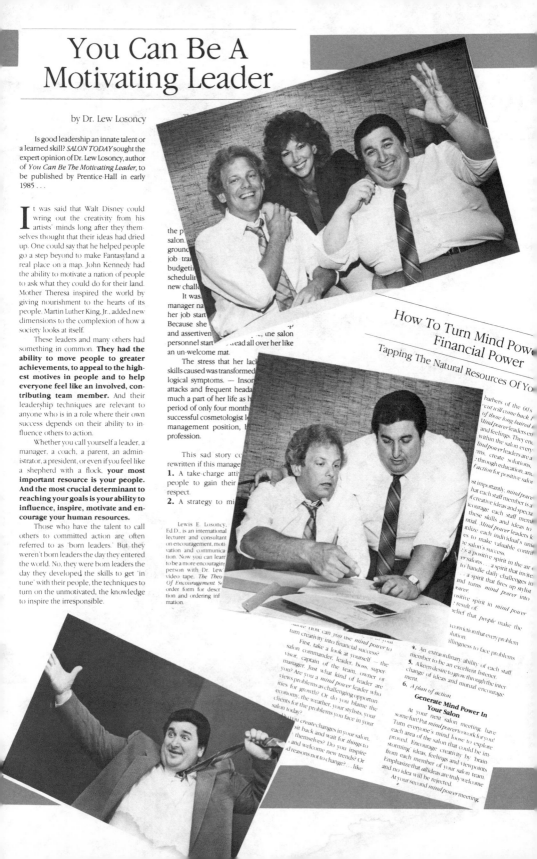

How To Turn Mind Pow... Financial Power
Tapping The Natural Resources Of Yo...

barbers of the 60's
...ent will come back f...
of those long haired...
Mind power leaders en...
and feelings. They enc...
within the salon every...
Mind power leaders are a...
...rms, create solutions...
...through education, an...
...f action for positive salon...

...st importantly, *mind powe*...
...hat each staff member is a...
...of creative ideas and specia...
...kourage each staff mem...
...these skills and ideas to...
...ntial. *Mind power* leaders k...
...es to make valuable contrit...
...e salon's success...
...'s a positive spirit in the air...
...versations . . . a spirit that invite...
...to handle daily challenges in...
...a spirit that fires up stylist...
...and turns *mind power* into...
...ower...

...ositive spirit in *mind power*...
...result of...
...elief that *people make the*...

...iconviction that every problem...
...olution...
...illingness to face problems...

4. An extraordinary ability of each staff member to be an excellent listener.
5. A keen desire to grow through the inter...change of ideas and mutual encourage...ment.
6. A plan of action.

Generate Mind Power In Your Salon

At your next salon meeting, have some fun! Put *mind power* to work for you! Turn everyone's *mind power* to work for you! each area of the salon that could be im...proved. Encourage creativity by brain...storming ideas, feelings and viewpoints from each member of your salon team. Emphasize that *all* ideas are truly welcome and no idea will be rejected.
At your second *mind power* meeting,

...low can you use *mind power* to...turn creativity into financial success?
First, take a look at yourself — the salon commander, leader, boss, super...visor, captain of the team, owner or manager. Just what kind of leader are you? Are you a *mind power* leader who views problems as challenging opportun...ities for growth? Or do you blame the economy, the weather, your stylists, your clients for the problems you face in your salon today?

...you *create* changes in your salon, ...sit back and wait for *things* to...themselves? Do you inspire...and welcome new trends? Or...d reasons *not* to change? . . . like

Learn To Communicate With Your Clients

Responsive —

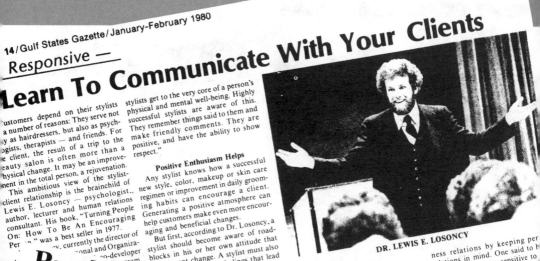

customers depend on their stylists for a number of reasons: They serve not only as hairdressers, but also as psychologists, therapists — and friends. For the client, the result of a trip to the beauty salon is often more than a physical change. It may be an improvement in the total person, a rejuvenation.

This ambitious view of the stylist-client relationship is the brainchild of Lewis E. Losoncy — psychologist, author, lecturer and human relations consultant. His book, "Turning People On: How To Be An Encouraging Person," was a best seller in 1977.

___, currently the director of ___ ___onal and Organiza___ ___o-developer ___am,

stylists get to the very core of a person's physical and mental well-being. Highly successful stylists are aware of this. They remember things said to them and make friendly comments. They are positive, and have the ability to show respect."

Positive Enthusiasm Helps

Any stylist knows how a successful new style, color, makeup or skin care regimen or improvement in daily grooming habits can encourage a client. Generating a positive atmosphere can help customers make even more encouraging and beneficial changes.

But first, according to Dr. Losoncy, a stylist should become aware of roadblocks in his or her own attitude that can prevent change. A stylist must also ___ aware of the feelings that lead ___rovement.

___ his attitude, the ___ly say, "I

in proper attitude, he said.

Stylists Need Empathy

Anyone who works with the public ___he feeling of being put down or ___ted by clients. Dr.

___ it's frustrating ___ a thank-you for ___eone. "But, that's ___ecommends "being ___ and sharing your ___at person. Empathy ___ share in another's ___ngs — opens the door ___ation." (He made a ___ion: "Empathy is under-___ client's world — sym-___g it!"

___cy gets positive feedback ___s who have improved busi-

ness relations by keeping per___ relations in mind. One said to h___ have become more sensitive to ___ and to negative mannerisms ___ such as walking away from clien___ I remember small things abo___ client, things important to the ___ handle difficult clients by using ___ approach, or simply by lis___ them."

The psychologist conclude___ ingredients can be taught to ___ in a short time. By saying ___ things at the right time ___ positive, a stylist can add to ___ affinity with his clients, ___ more effective when wo___ people."

DR. LEWIS E. LOSONCY

Psychologist warns against dwelling on life's mistakes

By CAROL NAPOLITANO
Press Staff Writer

LONG BEACH TOWNSHIP — The new year is here and with it comes the hope of a new beginning — a desire to pursue those resolutions you may have whispered to yourself as the clock struck midnight.

But, for some, the arrival of 1984 only marks the beginning of another 12 months of drudgery and depression. They suffer from sort of a hangover from life's problems and challenges which they think will never go away.

To them, Dr. Lewis E. Losoncy, psychologist, lecturer and author, says cheer up, there's hope.

Losoncy is the author of such works as "Turning People On," "The Encourage-___ent Book," "You Can Do It!" and "Think ___our Way to Success."

He is a former school guidance counselor and currently travels all over the U.S. and Canada speaking before teachers, students, psychologists, and business and industry representatives on how to create an air of enthusiasm and motivation in the lives and the lives of those around

___ there's one thing that people need ___of is the courage to be imperfect. The ___ing that keeps us from having the ___ is our disease of perfectionism,"
___soncy as he sat in the kitchen of his ___ Antioch Road in the High Bar
___ection here

___t of people believe that 'unless ___ect, I'm worthless," he said. ___ process of making big errors — ___ you can't be afraid to take

___ having a goal for the New ___lly important — something you ___k on next year and say that's ___ 1984," Losoncy said. "I just ___ufulfilled people. ___aid to have a full and happy ___ opt to take charge of your ___ this moment, right now, ___isputed fact — that is this is ___moment we'll ever have in

___it for something to happen ___ whole thing is up to me ___onsible for making your ___ birth sign, not the econo-___ not my parents, not my
___ said.

___ mistakes are beautiful ___ to learn from. People ___ out into the unknown ___ures of life and limit ___se of their fear of fail-

___ don't unpack your ___ trip on your adven-___goal," Losoncy said.

Sitting near his Long Beach ___ and lecturer, urges all to app

so many people's lives are boring and unhappy," he added. "Everyday try a new thing but don't expect to succeed rig. away."

And whatever you do — no matter how many times you fall, Losoncy said, have the courage to go on and never give up.

To make his point, Losoncy recited part of a poem he authored entitled "Sup-pose."

"Suppose the trees in giving up their leaves of fall felt that's all.

Suppose that higher times would never fall.

Well they would be wrong because life is too big not to have another song."

"If you have a negative attitude, everywhere you go you will see negatives.

Once you see things positively, everything in our world changes," he said.

Losoncy admits that encouraging and maintaining a positive attitude toward yourself is not easy and takes a lot of work.

"Feed your mind with good mind food, people," he said. "Stay away from negative people who give you advice...their advice obviously hasn't worked for them."

Losoncy said making amends with people you have not spoken to in years also helps a person become more productive.

"We've got to forgive and forget, not for what it will do for them, but what it will do for you" he said. "At the root of

"A passive attitude toward life is a dream.

With a bright smile and an engaging manner, he makes interviewing a breeze.

One question elicits colorful phraseology and scores of attention-getting quotes.

Losoncy has a way with people. In fact, when you get to the heart of the matter, people their quirks and their problems — provide Lo-soncy with a lucrative and interesting livelihood.

Losoncy is student of the human condition.

A grade-school teacher just a short decade ago, Losoncy went on to bigger and better things — a counselor, an administrator and professor of psychology at the Reading Area Community College and, ultimately, the author of a best-selling psychology book.

That book, "Turning People On: How to be an Encouraging Person," first published in 1977, is now in its seventh printing. More than 50,000 copies have been sold.

Losoncy, a Shillington resident, has followed that academic with another, "You Can Do It: How to Encourage Yourself."

He is currently on the lecture and seminar circuit, plugging the book and teaching organi-

---

Human Quirks, Hang-Ups

By DONNA REED
Eagle Staff Writer

Lew Losoncy is a reporter's dream.

zations and their members how to apply tenets discussed in the book to the reality of everyday life.

Originally, Losoncy said he wanted to title his book, "Get Off Your Can't." However, he said, Prentice-Hall, the publishers, rejected that title and came up with "You Can Do It."

Simple Philosophy

The philosophy of the brightly-written, easily comprehensible book, is simple, said its author.

"It is an anti-environment book," Losoncy said. "Your environment didn't make you who you are — you made yourself."

It also provides instruc-tions on taking the principles of encouragement and ap-plying those to one's self.

Losoncy, a Reading native who was graduated from Central Catholic High School and holds a doctorate in psy-chology, said his latest work encourages people to avoid using three basic words: should, ought and must.

"These are attempts to cre-ate a reality that doesn't ex-ist," Losoncy said. "Every-time we create a 'should' sit-uation, we create a misery."

An example? Losoncy men-tioned this:

"I'm not angry that I don't have a lot of money," he said. "I'm only angry when I be-

lieve I should have a lot of money."

Words To Avoid

There are other words and phrases to avoid, too, said Lo-soncy.

Those include if only, in my day and they say.

"Who the hell are 'they'?" Losoncy asked.

His recommendation for avoiding the use of these words and phrases is easy to remember: change sentences from the passive to active to avert placing blame on others for one's own condition at the moment.

Avoid blame and you cre-ate a greater chance for hap-piness, said Losoncy.

"At the root of all unhappi-ness is blaming," he said.

Losoncy also admonishes individuals not to restrict themselves to a particular self-image.

"We are all so complex,"

he said. "Everytime I see glimpses of the human possi-bility I am astounded.

"What limits us is what we choose to give importance to."

While counseling can give individuals better insight into their problems or hang-ups, said Losoncy, it is still up to the individual to pull himself out of depressions and take a more optimistic view of him-self and his surroundings.

Complainers and whiners tie up all their energies in useless ways.

"We'd like to shift the energies away and channel them in directions we hope will produce change." Lo-soncy said.

From his own vantage point, Losoncy would like to see the earth become a planet of CREEPS, filled with indi-viduals Constantly Ready to Encourage Every Person.

Author's Bag

The best way to ___ trend started, said ___ is for every individu___ a special someone___ for him/her all alo___

"One person ca___ the difference." ___ who heads the Re___ Institute for Per___ ganizational De___

He will be sp___ circuit around ___ several month___

Are You A People Builder?

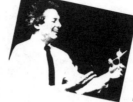

"If anything goes wrong, I, as the leader, will be blamed. So, I must live over my people's shoulders and watch them every step of the way to quickly point out their mistakes."

When a leader is under perceived threat, the stress experienced causes the person to react to errors in an exaggerated way. Instead of dealing with an error in a rational manner (let's correct it, or at least make the best of where we are right now), threatened leaders deal with the mistake irrationally (name calling, withdrawing, sulking, revenge).

Tension builds in an organization led by a threatened leader. People under threat live defensively. Defensive people can't create. The creation of new ideas is the answer to the mistakes. So, threatened leaders find themselves in a Catch 22 situation.

"It is my job as a leader to know more than anyone else. Since I am supposed to be the expert here, I can show my expertise best by criticizing, correcting, and spotting weakness."

Know it all leaders are threatened also, and try to cover up their feelings of inadequacy by believing the impossible notion that "I must know . . . more than anyone else here, since I am the one who knows the answer, my expertise is fine for a challenge. When I'm challenged by attempting . . . exposing . . .

"If you . . . get su . . . ageable . . ."

Some . . . spend mo . . . because th . . . rectors who . . . than the po . . . society funct . . . hasn't taken . . . cultural molo . . . ways of leading . . . to strengthen t . . .

"I assume a . . . Why should I f . . . ployees do wha . . . them? And anywe . . . they need to be m . . ."

The perfectionist . . . everyone will do a perf . . . need no recognition fo . . . achievements. But, failu . . . positives may lead to . . . People start to withdraw . . . slack off when they are ur . . . frontation may then be the . . . tion that appears appropria . . . been avoided by a more po . . . didn't assume perfection, bu . . . it and showed it. That's why th . . . leader never assumes that p . . . they are doing well.

Compensation: Is There An Easy Answer?

by Donald Scoleri

For more than three quarters of a century — from the Gibson girl topknot to today's nouveau punk haircut — the thorny question of how salon owners should pay their stylists has been the most controversial issue in the salon industry.

Some salon owners and stylists emphatically embrace commission, the most widely used method of payment, while others favor the growing trend toward salary. And sandwiched between both schools of thought are numerous alternatives of which many owners and stylists aren't even aware.

Frequently, worried salon owners will comment that their stylists don't understand financial management and persist in asking for higher commissions. In most cases, it's true that employees don't understand the slicing of the financial pie or how to read a profit and loss statement. This ignorance exists simply because no one has ever taken the time to explain financial statements to them. Granted, there is a lack of concern on the part of some owners and stylists, but many others do care and want to learn. It's a pity that the prevailing condition encourages confused thinking regarding the revenue salons bring in and the profits they share with their employees.

When considering alternative compensation systems — such as supply cost reimbursement, graduated sales quota, salary with incentives or bonuses, or a combination of all of these — the main question you must address is, *"What type of compensation will most satisfy the needs . . . staff?"*

en you observe uplifting 'ders, whether they be agers, parents, coaches, you consistently see a nt present in their

g leaders spend 'development success of ed to the eople

lves ted d

In some salo . . . issue b . . .

It's all how you look at things, says speaker

By MIKE BOYER

It's not the way life is that affects you, but the way you choose to look at it, says Lewis Losoncy, a professor of positive attitude.

"The key is how we choose to look at things," says Losoncy, a teacher, author and lecturer, who is in Elmira this week to conduct a two-day seminar using his ideas for the Chemung County Labor Management Committee.

The first session for about 60 representatives of local labor and management will be held this afternoon at the Elmira Holiday Inn.

Basically Losoncy emphasizes looking at things in a positive rather than negative light, and assuming responsibility for life rather than blaming others.

Emphasizing the negative in human relationships is a self-fulfilling prophecy, he said.

For example he cited the teacher who was constantly calling a student stupid and when the student failed asked was asked why the student failed "How do you expect me to act, I'm stupid."

A professor of psychology at Reading, Pa., Area Community College as well as author of a book — "Turning People On — How To Be An Encouraging Person," Losoncy said his seminar emphasizes positive thinking.

"When a counselor stopped me in the hall one day and said, 'You have a fantastic talent,' he said. 'You have a real talent for getting the nuns (who taught at the school) to swear at you.'

"Now if you could just turn that talent around and use it in a different way.'

"That turned me around. I went to college," he said. Later as a college admissions director, Losoncy said he saw students failing because they had negative attitudes about themselves."

What emerged, he said was what he calls the "science of encouragement," using what he admits are commonsense approaches to motivate people.

"My philosophy is that psychology doesn't belong in the classroom but in the community."

With that in mind Losoncy said he spends much of his time traveling around the country explaining his concepts to groups ranging from hair stylists to prison officials.

Losoncy says he asks people to focus on strengths rather than weaknesses. People assume a negative attitude because it is the easiest way to say "I can't" than to try, he said.

"I encourage people to be more task-involved. It's much easier for a person to be negative because it tells you there's an alternative. Success is only a fringe benefit," he said.

"Most people don't take a chance and wish they had."

Losoncy says he believes most of what is described as emotional illness

is the result of negative attitude.

Another element in his philosophy, Losoncy said requires people to face reality.

"Stop expecting anybody to give us anything and that life is fair. Take responsibility for your own life. Stop blaming others and start living life.

As part of the process which facilitates better communication, Losoncy says he asks those who he works with

to "get out of their world and things as others see them."

Losoncy says the belief tha . . . can be motivated out of fea . . . ized in such books an . . . through intimidation, br . . . the person doing the in . . . enough over the . . .

"I say the most . . . motivating thro . . . idation but thr . . . and rewarding th . . .

TALKING POSITIVE — Lewis Losoncy, a Reading, Pa., psychologist and author, discusses his belief in positive attitude. He is in Elmira this week to conduct a seminar for the Chemung County Labor Management Committee.

Local

Lewis Losoncy
DOES YOUR SUCCESS DEPEND . . .
PERFORMANCE . . .
OF OTHERS? . . .
IF SO, YOU CAN BE . . .

Motivati . . . Lead . . .

BRIEFING ON PR . . .
UPLIFTING APPROA . . .
RESPONSIBLE, MOTI . . .
EMPLOYEES . . .
ON CHILDREN, STU . . .
FOR THE FIRST TIM . . .
LIST OF LEADER . . .
BEHAVIORS THAT MA . . .
SAID MOTIVATED T . . .

is an internation . . .
agement, to any . . .
newest book . . .
approaches to . . .
ur business . . .
you kno . . .
o your . . .
iques . . .
for

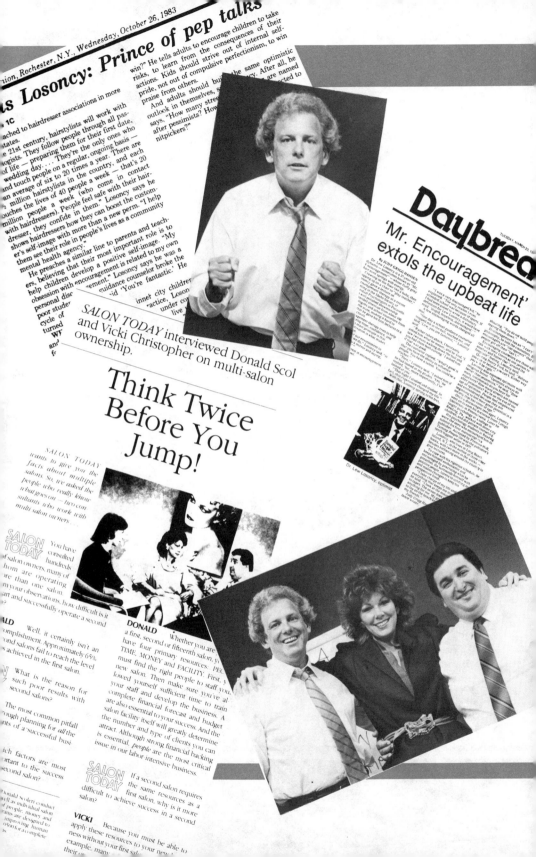

as Losoncy: Prince of pep talks

1C

ached to hairdresser associations in more
states.

e 21st century, hairstylists will work with
ogists. They follow people through all pas-
of life.... They're the only ones who
wedding day.... touch people on a regular, ongoing basis —
an average of six to 20 times a year. There are
million hairstylists in the country, and each
ouches the lives of 40 people a week — that's 20
million people a week (who come in contact
with hairdressers). People feel safe with their hairdresser, they confide in them." Losoncy says he
shows hairdressers how they can boost the customer's self-image with more than a new perm. "I help
them see their role in people's lives as a community
mental health agency."

He preaches a similar line to parents and teachers, believing that their most important role is to
help children develop a positive self-image. "My
obsession with encouragement is related to my own
personal dis-   'ement." Losoncy says he was a
poor stude-   guidance counselor broke the
cycle of   id 'You're fantastic. He
turned   inner city children
W   ractice, Loson
an   under co
f   live

win?" He tells adults to encourage children to take
risks, to learn from the consequences of their
actions. Kids should strive out of internal self-
pride, not out of compulsive perfectionism, to win
praise from others.

And adults should b   the same optimistic
outlook in themselves, s   are named
says, "How many stre   cted to
after pessimists? How
nitpickers?"

SALON TODAY interviewed Donald Scol
and Vicki Christopher on multi-salon
ownership.

Think Twice Before You Jump!

SALON TODAY
wants to give you the
facts about multiple
salons. So, we asked the
people who really know
what goes on — two con-
sultants who work with
multi-salon owners...

SALON TODAY   You have
consulted hundreds
of salon owners, many of
hom are operating
ore than one salon.
m your observations, how difficult is it
art and successfully operate a second

ALD   Well, it certainly isn't an
omplishment. Approximately 65%
ond salons fail to reach the level
s achieved in the first salon.

V   What is the reason for
7   such poor results with
second salons?

The most common pitfall
ough planning for *all the*
nts of a successful busi-

ch factors are most
ortant to the success
second salon?

ould So deri conduct
well as individual salon
f people, money and
ants are designed to
improving human
potion for a complete

DONALD   Whether you are
a first, second or fifteenth salon, y
have four primary resources: PEO
TIME, MONEY and FACILITY. First, y
must find the right people to staff you
new salon. Then make sure you've allowed yourself sufficient time to train
your staff and develop the business. A
complete financial forecast and budget
are also essential to your success. And the
salon facility itself will greatly determine
the number and type of clients you can
attract. Although strong financial backing
is essential, *people* are the most critical
issue in our labor-intensive business.

VICKI   If a second salon requires
the same resources as a
first salon, why is it more
difficult to achieve success in a second
salon?

Because you must be able to
apply these resources to your new
ness without your first sal
example, many
their

Daybrea

TUESDAY, MARCH 20, 1

'Mr. Encouragement' extols the upbeat life

By JUDY GRIGG HANSEN

Dr. Lew Losoncy optimist

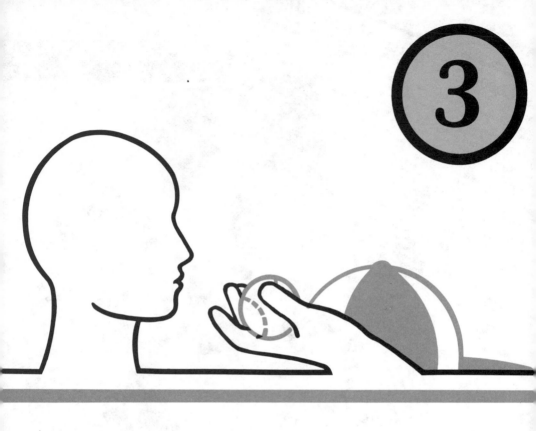

The New Psy-Cosmetologist: A Dedicated Team Player

FROM "ME THINKING"
TO "WE THINKING"

A dramatic transition has been taking place in the social structure of the salon. Whereas in the 1950s and 1960s stylists, then called "operators," needed to be concerned primarily with themselves, salons staffed with **psy-cosmetologists in the 1980s are faced with the challenge of making salon decisions based on what's best for *everyone*.** We are witnessing the blossoming from "me" to "we" thinking. The people in the "we power" salons know that their overall success is related to the cooperation, commitment, and efforts of all team members.

This attitude of power in numbers is consistent with the findings of psychobiologists, who study animal behavior. Animals ban together to make their colonies stronger against attacks by predators. And although one animal couldn't survive an attack from the environment, many animals united together with a purpose are more likely to resist an aggressive advance. Interestingly, the more the animals work together with a common purpose, the stronger each one becomes. Indeed Joshua Liebman wrote in *Hope for Man* that evidence suggests it is not survival of the fittest, as Darwin claimed, but rather that nature is governed by the principle of "cooperate or die."

"We power" salons recognize that same fact, that the more the team players are united by a common purpose, the more power each one has individually. Total team-involved salons not only affect the attitudes and successes of each of their members, but also have an impact on society itself, because the one who benefits from this positive team atmosphere is the client.

Individuals of the 1950s and 1960s

The professional salon industry has experienced far-reaching changes in the period from 1950 to the current time. The barber shops and beauty parlors of the 1950s, as you recall, were neighborhood based, composed of one or two barbers or operators. Being neighborhood centered, they did their styling in a localized area, drawing father-son, mother-daughter traffic. Competition was minimal, because malls, strip centers, and centralized salons were rare. The cutter would see clients on a weekly or bi-weekly basis and would build his or her security around this guarantee. The professional in a one-person shop functioned in total isolation from everything and everybody. The process of growth fell almost totally on individuals, and they were capable of succeeding that way in that time in the evolution of our society. Teamwork was not an issue that one had to address on the road to success.

Cliques of the 1970s

With the growth of the industry in the 1970s, salon size increased to keep pace with growing needs. All of a sudden for the first time in history, the salon had a number of people under its roof. The salon now crystalized into a "social structure" with all of its joys and problems. For the most part, cutting shops weren't prepared. Imagine the complications involved in the change from a one-person salon to a three-person salon. It's like two other people moving into another person's house. People tend to take sides. Hence in many salons, cliques were formed, binding people together against other people.

Also, competitiveness that didn't exist in the one-person shop became an everyday fact of life. Judgment of the stylist's work increased. The consumer could now compare his or her stylist's talents with the work of others in the same shop. Competitiveness was heightened. In all of this competitiveness, an in-crowd, out-crowd feeling emerged and some salon personnel worked *against* rather than *with* each other.

But change was on the horizon. The new psy-cosmetologists of the twenty-first century were waiting in the embryonic stage. From a nucleus of progressive individuals and cliques would emerge the offspring, the salon team players.

Salon Team Players
of the 21st Century

The new psy-cosmetologists are the far-sighted individuals who see the whole salon as being more than just the sum of its parts. They believe that it is much more productive and healthier to work in an atmosphere of mutual respect and trust. They are above the belief that they are in competition and instead highlight the importance of cooperation.

They are people developers. They enlist the resources and assets of each and every team member and encourage the development of each member's fullest potential. The new psy-cosmetologists have an inherent sense that as the team grows, so will they grow, because the strengthened team has more resources to satisfy each member's needs.

Team power or "we power" means that everyone is a contributing member who is an important part of the whole. When one stylist is having a rough time, everyone pulls together to find a way to resolve the issue, because they all know that when they have tough times, others will do the same. The team attitude makes the difference. More and more progressive salon owners are looking for these team players to be part of their salons.

Team Attitude
Makes the Difference

A personal friend of ours from Vancouver, Canada, Geoffrey L., says, *My hiring policy is totally developed around the applicant's attitude toward self and team. I can train people in technical skills. If they have an open mind and a positive attitude joining our team-oriented salon, we can usually work on the other modifications. However, if someone has that "I'll do it my way" feeling or "You can't teach me anything" attitude, we don't stand for it. We have worked long and hard to develop this concept, and the team realizes what we have, and we want to keep it. The team atmosphere has been established, and we're not going to give it up for a single individual.*

ADVANTAGES OF
TEAM POWER SALONS

Pride

Why does Geoffrey's staff want to protect what they have worked so hard to develop? *Pride.* Team power salons do not become team salons without a lot of sweat, tears, and hard work. This develops a sense of pride in their accomplishments. They know that the reason they have succeeded when many others have given up is because of their effort and dedication. They are living, breathing examples of people who are enjoying their fruits and rewards after stumbling many times, getting up and trying again and again until they succeeded.

Combined Efforts

Just by logical reasoning, team salons make common sense. **By working as a team, these people can and do accomplish more than any single entity.** It's just good sense working together, because when you multiply the efforts of a group, look at the long-term benefits that everyone receives.

Being in Tune with Society

Finally, and most importantly, team salons are in tune with the Human Revolution and thus are becoming the most popular choices for a selective public. The team salon offers multi-options, multi-services, and flexible hours to draw the clients of today. But, the big draw is the special psy-cosmetologists who have cultivated their skills of sensitivity to become the well-rounded professionals who the client demands of the team salon. Team players know what they have to do, and they do it.

THE ULTIMATE GIFTS OF TEAM POWER SALONS

Gifts of Caring in a Warm Environment

The salon team atmosphere provides the richest soil in which to grow and develop. Each team member has a true concern for his or her coworkers' needs and desires. Psy-cosmetologists do not have to shoulder their salon problems by themselves. The caring atmosphere in the "we power" salons helps to resolve problems. The psy-cosmetologist not only understands and cares about his or her own clients, but also expresses the same concern for peers' clients. In team power salons, stylists don't have to fight over clients. The goal is to have contented clients, so whoever can fulfill a need is the one who performs the service. There's a healthy, comfortable environment, which is a gift of the team player to the client. **There are fewer underlying negative feelings among the personnel in team power salons because of this mutual understanding** of working together. The results are seen clearly by the client. The client's return visit is the gift to the salon personnel.

Gifts of a Second Family

At a staff meeting we attended, one stylist bubblingly shared one of the benefits of their salon. Rose said, *Where I worked before, I would go into long periods of boredom. In our salon however, there is always something happening, and there is electricity in the air. We are always going around trying to lift each other's spirits. It's just never dull here.* (She laughed.) *With all these creative people working around you, how could you ever get bored? Someone is always saying, "Hey, look at this new color design," or 'Watch this new perm wrap," or "Get into this heavy looking cut." It's like party time with each client. We're all involved each time a client is designed and everyone makes a fuss. It's just neat. You can just imagine how the clients feel!*

Dennis spoke up and supported Rose. The tall, dark-haired enthusiast added, *What makes me feel good is how everyone around here keeps telling me I can do it when I get down. They won't let me give up! They say successful people just keep trying until they accomplish their goals!*

Then, this gentle voice softly added, *The specialness that I feel is that we give of ourselves freely to each other without being forced or intimidated to do so.* Cindy continued, *As you know, I come from a bad past, and my life started to come together when I became a cosmetologist. Working with you is like having the family I never had.* As eyes filled up with tears of love, the warmth was like a strong burning fire on a snowy winter night. These flames would not go out easily. These were flames of human togetherness.

Finally, after a few moments of silence, a heavyset gentleman said, *We all feel what Cindy feels, but it is time to go on, so we can keep this spirit going forward.* The owner, Dan, started to move on to the next business topic and looked out at those faces and said, *What the hell, let's call it a night and enjoy ourselves.* **The ultimate gift of love and caring in team salons gives people a feeling of being in the presence of a second family, a family that they are with for almost as many hours as they are with their first families.**

Gifts to the Client

In some salons, we have observed salon members introducing their clients to other team members' clients. This creates a sense of ease for clients because they get the opportunity to develop new relationships. This contact also provides a pleasant social climate for clients. It's essential in getting clients to feel at ease in the salon. These relationships many times continue outside the salon. Lifelong friendships have developed from salon introductions. What a gift! And when you consider the frequent contact of six to fifty times a year in a salon, the salon really is a social center in society.

Gifts to the Community

One of the most touching stories told to us was by a Haddonfield, New Jersey salon owner named Tony S. One of Tony's objectives was to stimulate ongoing community activity. The staff, a cohesive team, discussed ways of getting more involved in community activities to provide long-term help for the less fortunate through salon efforts.

After brainstorming for ideas, the salon team came to the conclusion that people who have disabilities don't want to be pitied. They want the same respect and concern anyone else receives. Tony and his psy-cosmetologists reached out by making people with disabilities aware that they were wanted and welcomed, not just on certain days or special days, but whenever they chose to frequent the salon.

Tony commented, *We like to have three or four promotions yearly for special organizations and turn the proceeds of the day over to the organizations.* Tony proudly shared the fact that all staff members give freely of their time and energy. *We are all well rewarded by the support we receive all year long from the entire community,* the sensitive owner explained. *Our salon people just want to give a little back.*

Tony and his group of psy-cosmetologists truly exemplify the team power salon. **The gift of giving is part of the twenty-first-century team salon; giving of oneself to become part of something much bigger than oneself,** which is a *team.*

The four-star hair salon is housed with team members who desire to serve their clients to the optimum. Who are these receptionists, cleansing technicians, stylists, perm and color specialists, and skin care technicians who are team-oriented? What special tools and skills do these members possess? Mainly they have an awareness that their own personal success hinges on their willingness to interact responsibly and positively with other team members.

THE RECEPTIONIST

I (Donald Scoleri) had the pleasure of attending a receptionist training symposium in 1982 in Cherry Hill, New Jersey. The seminar was to further develop the skills of the receptionist. From the moment I arrived I sensed a special attitude in the room, the way the receptionists were dressed, their friendly smiles, and their warm introductions to each other.

The lecturer made his opening remarks and then asked a few questions of the participants. *When you hear the word "receptionist," what does it mean to you?* Surprisingly, several hands went up at once. An attractive, mature woman rose from her chair. She turned to the group and, almost without speaking a word, commanded attention.

Stage Setters

The woman introduced herself as Linda and went on to say, *We are the first natural link to a successful salon visit. We represent the entire salon's concept, and we have the responsibility to present the most professional picture possible. Our clients start painting a mental picture the moment we answer the telephone. When they first enter the salon, they draw a first impression. A warm, friendly attitude is essential for a positive picture to develop for the client. We set the stage for what will follow. The stage can be unpleasant or it can be pleasant. Either way, we can create an attitude within customers that they carry with them throughout their whole visit with us.*

Image Makers and PR Ambassadors

Another hand went up. Like an excited student who had the right answer, "Bubbles" stood up. It was my feeling that Bubbles was her nickname because she just "bubbles" over with enthusiasm. Her precious smile covered her entire face. Her youthfulness seemed to disappear in her opening words.

First, I love being a receptionist. I work with the greatest group of people. To me the word receptionist means creating a lasting positive impression, so when our clients leave they have no reason to think about going anywhere else. We are the image makers. *My stylists call me the Public Relations Ambassadoress. I know that if I do positive things for the client, it will help each member of the staff.*

Organizers

Robin said, *My boss has so many things to do in a day. He designs hair, helps the staff, handles business matters, and I guess I could go on and on. To help, I organize a written agenda of priorities for him. I won't bother him with foolish phone calls or calls that could be handled later. I respect his time. I try to anticipate his needs and help. I know he really appreciates when I help organize his daily schedule.* So, one way that a receptionist helps the team is through organizing.

Bookers, Pacers, and Problem Preventers

Kathy, another receptionist, added, *I know it's really important for the stylists to have their appointments booked correctly. I am a stickler about that. One poor booking can foul up a stylist's whole day. Also, I try to help with another area. I know that sometimes stylists lose sight of the time, because they are so involved artistically. So, we have a code word worked out, and I just walk by and communicate our code word to let them know we are running late and try to do so without making the clients feel they are being rushed. We all want the clients in the styling chairs to think and feel that that's their special time, and it is! And finally, the thing I think stylists appreciate more than anything else is when we understand the pressures they are under on a daily basis and help prevent problems before they occur.* A receptionist who is a team player strives for accurate books, paces the salon, and anticipates and deals with problems.

Easers of Pressure on New Team Members

Tina piggybacked, *Our salon is really growing, so I had a chance to work with a lot of new stylists this year. Their first year in the salon can be a difficult one. They feel strange and are hit with many new things in a short period of time. My cleansing technician, co-designer, and assistants look to me to help make the new person feel at home and part of the team, because they themselves don't always have the time. The receptionist is the most logical one to help out in the first few weeks of a new stylist's arrival.*

First Ladies of the Salon

Later on in the day, the group leader observed that his eyes had been opened by the extensive education receptionists must go through; answering telephones, booking appointments, controlling inventory, handling cash drawers, making schedules, setting up staff meetings, promoting services and products, regulating traffic, and on and on to an almost endless job description about the salon's "first lady."

Receptionists have a difficult role because they do not start with a license as do stylists and other team members. They must learn all the facts of the industry and understand thoroughly enough to be able to explain to clients how these services can best enhance their appearances. They are called on to be the links between all the processes of communication that occur in the salon. **Receptionists are the beginning and the ending links. They must have the foresight to anticipate, not only the clients' needs, but also the staff's needs, and yet carry out their regular duties effectively.**

We'll end this praise of the receptionist as a salon team member with a dramatic story we heard from a receptionist who exemplifies the cream of the crop in client caring.

Winning Clients Over

Joan S. shared, *I was working in a new salon, and we were located inside a mini-mall. Suddenly, a bicycle stopped outside of our front window, and a very mature woman got off the bike and came into the salon. At first appearance, I was a bit startled. But I pulled my composure together quickly. She was a short woman with two long ponytails hanging down the middle of her back, wearing a slightly tarnished dress and no shoes.*

I asked politely, "May I help you?"

"Do you do wash and sets, and will you take me now since I don't want to wait?"

"Yes, we do," I said with a smile. "Our salon will be happy to have you as a client." I noticed her sneakers on the handlebars of the bike outside. "Would you like to bring your bike inside? Then you can get your sneakers if you like."

She said, "Are you going to force me to put my sneakers on?"

I said, "No." I saw a sigh of relief cross her weathered face.

"Then, I'll put them on. But, how long am I going to have to wait to get my hair done?"

"We have an opening right now and we would be happy to style your hair."

"I guess you are going to want to cut my hair," she stated while nervously running her fingers through her hair.

"No, not necessarily," I responded. *"How do you feel about your length of hair?"*

Shrugging her shoulders, pulling and tugging on her hair like a small child, she stumbled to find the right words, then said with a curled lip, *"I like it long!"*

"Then I'll tell your stylist not to cut your hair. We'll shampoo and set your hair for you, or would you like us to rebraid it?"

The lady, trying not to smile, said, *"I can braid my own hair."* With a tone of challenge in her voice, she said, *"Can't they do something different?"*

Her salon experience began, and soon she left with a smile and a new hairdo. The little woman with the tough attitude, tattered clothes, and unkempt appearance turned out to be one of the most influential women in town. She spread the news of her acceptance of this salon through the town, because of Joan's understanding of her special needs. Joan was a First Lady in a salon.

Rallying Point of the Salon Team

The example of this very special woman, Joan S., points out dramatically the important effect the receptionist has on the salon's success. The interactions that occur between the receptionist and other staff members are complex, and in many cases the receptionist is the rallying point of the salon. With multi-antenna communication sensors, **the receptionist has the ability to pull the salon together when the call for action arises.** As Rose pointed out, the receptionist is the first natural link.

Good receptionists are stage setters, image makers, public relations ambassadors, organizers, accurate bookers, salon pacers, problem preventors, easers of pressure on new team members, and first ladies of the salon.

THE CLEANSING TECHNICIAN

The client's journey through the salon is now guided by his or her second contact, the cleansing technician. With precision teamwork well planned in advance, the transition from receptionist to cleansing technician can be a smooth experience for the paying client. The cleansing technician's numerous responsibilities are another important part of the client's visit to the salon.

In many cases, the cleansing technician's deeds are overlooked by the client, but his or her part on the team is essential. The cleansing technician frequently has to work extra hard to gain the respect of the client because of his or her youthfulness, which tends to be equated with inexperience. If the management and the stylists show respect for the cleansing technician, this attitude rubs off on the client.

Everyone knows how therapeutic a scalp massage can be. The cleansing technician must try to get the client into a relaxed frame of mind in preparation for the next experience, the actual cut, color, or perm. **Client relaxation is a direct result of having confidence in the cleansing technician.**

Why shouldn't they have confidence in me? Joann asks. *I completed cosmetology school, put in all my necessary hours and requirements, and passed my state boards of cosmetology. That was months of hard work, day after day of tedious procedures, of learning everything from a pincurl, to learning every bone in the body. From finger waves to perm waves, from nail coloring to hair coloring.*

We do not take our responsibilities lightly. Just the other day, Michael, one of our stylists, said I was doing a great job in choosing the right shampoo for his clients' hair, and he was real pleased to know that I was there. I have my license right above where I work. Often, Michael will tell me what shampoo he would like me to use, but I explain to the clients all the benefits that will magnify the positive aspects of their hair. Why shouldn't clients have confidence in us, with all of our training?

Pride in Knowledge

You could just smell the pride that Bob C., a recent graduate, took in knowing every single shampoo and conditioner and what capabilities each product had. *I love the science of our products, and I love pointing out the practicality of them to the clients. I think our stylists and clients alike trust me,* Bob shared proudly. *We can help them because we know what we're doing. You can't frighten people about hair and scalp situations. Show them the positive attributes of their hair, and they will let you help them.* Bob concluded on the sensitive note that, *It won't be long and I'll be styling and I'll remember to help our cleansing technicians.*

A Time to Learn: Investment in the Future

Often, the cleansing technician's role is very challenging, explained Linda P., *because we're needed to help in so many* areas. We seem to be scrutinized by the clients more closely than the stylist who has been around longer and is established. Sometimes, new team members have difficulty grasping the big picture. This can be their proving grounds, to themselves and to the clients. Actually, a cleansing technician communicates with more clients in a day than a stylist does. What a way to get to know your clients' likes and dislikes! Think about it! We learn from the importance of every step that occurs to our clients. We set the stage for a pleasurable experience for our clients.

Communication Through Touch

Touch is an integral part of the appointment, starting with the shampoo. The client starts to escape the reality of the outside world and think totally about himself or herself while enjoying the relaxing comforts of the cleansing technician's skills. A refreshing, dry, clean towel with a pleasant fragrance is placed around the client's neck. Then a cutting cloth or cape is added to fit snugly. The client's head is gently laid back into the shampoo bowl. The cleansing technician runs his or her fingers through the client's hair before allowing the water to throb onto the scalp and hair fibers! Then the delicate, thick lather of the shampoo cascades onto the client's hair. The fragrant shampoo is gently massaged throughout the scalp area and into every single hair fiber.

The Magic Moment

The cleansing technician continued the explanation of the shampooing process. The cleansing technician's ten fingers work like mini-electric "massagers" on the client's scalp, almost putting him or her into a trance. While rinsing the first lather out, the cleansing technician can feel the tenseness in the client's body dissipate, and a gentle smile appears almost secretively so as not to give away how much he or she enjoys the massage. The client moves his or her head into position for the second lathering, anticipating where the next massage movement will come from. Those five minutes of cleansing and scalp massaging can make the difference in the overall success of that visit. Whether shampooing or assisting the colorist or the permist, the role of the cleansing technician is an important one in the overall success of the salon.

Their Place on the Team

Linda described it this way: I was in charge of the cleansing area for about six months. It was Herb's third day on the job.

Fridays in the salon can be frightening to a new employee who is not accustomed to them. Herb found himself being pushed to do three or four things at once. He looked like a puzzle coming apart. Herb's anger was very obvious, and he had the clients and the other cleansing technicians upset with his mumbling under his breath.

Realizing what Herb was going through, I asked him to come to the dispensary with me. I then went back and calmed down the clients, had one of the cleansing technicians finish up, and I went to talk to Herb.

Normally, our receptionist is real good at handling this situation, but she was so busy, I took on the task. I said, "Herb, I understand how you feel. You're feeling confused and frustrated right now. You're being asked to spread yourself out, sometimes like peanut butter!"

Herb forced a smile, trying to hold back his emotion. "I heard the barrage you were hit with this morning: shampoo, fold towels, bring people back here, sweep the floor, mix a color, get the perm rods, rinse a color off, go get lunch. I guess you feel like you're not important."

Herb's head was bent down, and he was shuffling his feet. Our eyes met, and there was a mutual understanding without speaking a word. Herb's body straightened and I knew Herb had jumped one of the hurdles of his occupation.

Reality Sets In

"Do you realize that without us, this place might stop in its tracks?" I said kiddingly. Herb's smile was like finding a lost friend! Herb said, "You're right!" "All that activity that's going on, every team member will show you and tell you how they feel. They have been saying it, you haven't been hearing it because you became frustrated so quickly. Herb, you are here because we all have confidence in you. We are responsible for important functions that occur in this salon. We keep the entire salon network moving systematically. That's how we get so popular with the entire clientele so quicky. Everybody gets to share a little bit of us."

"Someday, Herb, you and I will be styling those clients." Just then, the receptionist came back and said, "Hey, you know this place can't run with you two hiding out here. Linda, I thought you were going to come up and tell us when the last shampoo was completed. I depend on you to do that for me." We all knew what we had to do. As Linda so beautifully reflected, the cleansing technician's role has a direct effect on the salon team members.

The Vital Link

Cleansing technicians are the first people to touch clients. They set the styling stage by helping to build positive anticipation for the clients' cuts, perms or color. They must understand the benefits of specific shampoos and conditioners, must go through a growing period in the salon, and finally must be part of the team.

THE COSMETOLOGIST OR BARBER-STYLIST

Like painters and sculptors, hair designers, through a repetitive process, develop excellence in their craft that evolves into a profession. The educational process of hair designers just begins when they graduate and receive their first degree, which is a license to practice professional cosmetology or barber-styling. **In the Human Revolution, the ultimate designers must not only continue to develop their technical skills, but also find the delicate balance of "people" skills.** In forecasting their future, it is clear that an ongoing maturation of technical skills will be essential. But, as we look to the designer of the twenty-first century, the need for human awareness is also crucial.

Psy-cosmetologists stay enthusiastic and well prepared for the constant changes that are occurring in the world, especially the ones that affect their clientele. The talent designers share with their clients creates the magic of cosmetic beauty outside, and inner beauty from within. This next story reflects yet another skill of the psy-cosmetologist in the quest for excellence.

Giving Freely to Other Team Members

Troy T. told us how he shares his haircutting skills with all the newest staff members. *I remember when I started out, how eager I was to learn. But unfortunately, there was no one who wanted to help me. Finally, the pressure to grow quickly with no guidance really hurt me early in my career. I learned the hard way, through trial and error, and that is a traumatic way to learn when you are working on people.*

So, I try to give guidance to the young designers. I get a big thrill seeing the cleansing technicians and assistant designers finishing their day and waiting to start our workshop so they can cut some hair. The cleansing technicians and assistants help me all day with my responsibilities. As the designers are styling during the day, you can sense the assistants' fantasies about what they would do if they were working on the clients. You can almost hear their thoughts that "someday, hair, you will be all mine!"

Tony continued, It's just professional courtesy to help other staff members. When they are designing hair full-time, each person they do is part of me walking out the door. Each of us affects the other person's future growth!

Developing Communicative Skills

Sitting in the Philadelphia airport one Saturday afternoon, we entered into a conversation with a stylist from Delaware. Larry was a smooth, well-dressed haircutter who started telling us about the salon and his spirited past. When I graduated from cosmetology school, I was wet behind the ears, but I thought I knew everything. I was a hotshot and I had all the right answers. What I was really doing was covering up my insecurities. I was a cocky kid with some talent, but had a hard time relating and trusting people. My ways always seemed the better ways. Larry told us he was on his way down to Atlanta to attend a special communications seminar, and that his boss was paying for the entire trip. Larry stopped for a second, and you could tell that the next words would have special meaning.

Giving Back to the Salon Team

A big, friendly smile appeared, and at the same time, Larry took on a taller stature. I had to realize what I didn't know. Now, I'm both stylist and communications director for our salon. My boss is so pleased that I have taken these responsibilities off his shoulders.

When asked how he became stylist and communications director, Larry explained, Stu was responsible for the transition. He saw the raw talent in my cutting ability, but more important, he saw my human qualities. I made a promise to Stu that, because of this help, I would become the best stylist his salon had ever seen. Hence, I slowly worked my way up the ranks. My comments were that each and every person in our salon would have the best training and knowledge available to them. I finally realized that to be truly productive, they needed all the resources we could offer. I wanted to do this for myself and Stu.

I never realized how communications would monopolize my learning for a long, long time. I slowly learned the needs of Stu, the staff, and of course the clients. I became aware of the real world and the people in it. The feeling I get inside brings goose bumps to my body.

As we sat and listened to Larry, we felt his pride in how he grew and how he helped other team members grow. We knew even in that brief airport encounter that we were in the presence of a real psy-cosmetologist.

Combining the Ultimate Cutter with the Ultimate Specialist

When the artistry of a dynamic haircutter is combined with the talents of a perm or coloring specialist, we experience a whole new salon creation. As Joe M. pointed out, *The most exciting time I spend creating is when one of our specialists and myself work together with a client. We love originating the total look for a client, combining both of our minds. The dimensional design of our perm, color, and the finishing touches with the essence of skin care and a new cosmetic application, the total look with just one client generates a stimulation for other staff members and clients alike.* Joe went on to say that with more and more working women, the salon consultation was more in demand. **The consultation guarantees fulfilling the individual's needs.**

From the Victorian Age to the Total Look

Joe added, *The total-look concept has caught on quite well with our male and female clientele. Males have to be encouraged a little more, but their looks are just as important in the working and social world. We have come out of the Victorian Age and are doing what makes us look and feel good. We, as professional designers, are the information center for our clients. Who better than us understands the client and his or her lifestyle?*

With the blending of our talents, clients see that we are working together to enhance their appearance. They become very comfortable with this complement of attention and skills. Many clients are sheepish about their feelings because they have been put down or intimidated at other salons. We explain to our clients that they are here to have fun, to feel good about what's happening and that absolutely nothing will ever be done to them without them feeling comfortable with the end result. If they are not content, we will take the time until they are. Our motto is:

"Not one snip of hair, nor one perm rod, nor one stroke of color until you're ready! Then we can enjoy the beauty experience together!"

The hair designer is working in conjunction with the other specialists in the salon to develop an atmosphere of confidence and good will and to create a long, healthy bond.

A Silent Experience that Spoke Loudly

A most exciting experience happened to us while on a lecturing trip. We had occasion to watch a Japanese artistic team perform their artistry. The music was the soft sounds of their ancestry playing in the background. The audience waited with anticipation as the lights were lowered and the spotlights fell on this group of foreign intrigue.

A voice came over the speakers, gently blending with the music, and announced, *Please sit back and relax. We want you to enjoy and learn everything you desire. However, we need your cooperation. Please put your total concentration on center stage, and you will learn everything you desire about these designs.* The audience became slightly restless, but the up-tempo of the music engulfed them as the artists whirled around their respective models.

The Experience Begins

Opening their gowns, they started taking out their cutlery, which glistened from the spotlights. The audience gasped. They put their cutlery down, but the audience seemed to sense the specialness of the hour. As they delicately combed through each model's hair, there seemed to be a rhythm with the team, yet each one exposed his or her own intensity in the situation. They handled the hair fiber as though holding a small, delicate baby between their fingers. Painstakingly, every snag and snarl was released from its bondage. With almost magical quickness, they twirled the hair, quickly creating a design just by twisting it!

The audience applauded, then moved closer to the edges of their chairs, and you could sense the excitement. There were many young hairdesigners in that audience, and their eyes danced with anticipation of the next creation.

A Silent Performance

Almost simultaneously, the artistic team started to section each model's hair, with still not a word from the performers. Yet, the rapport and communication had been well established without verbal communication. As the audience's eyes danced from model to model to watch all three haircuts at the same time, they finally relaxed and adjusted to the fact that very few words would be spoken on this day.

The team worked with laser-like accuracy in cleaning out each parting before the scissors were raised. The final decision was near. Each artist combed through each section over and over again until the flow seemed right.

With no indecision whatsoever, the scissors glided through the sections of hair, and it fell gently to the floor. The artists, almost as if asking without asking, looked at the audience, pointed to the hair, and repeated the same step over and over again.

The artists made sure to be out of the audience's way as they performed their wizardry with scissors and comb. Molding the fiber, moving it around, placing the hair, and then replacing it over and over again. The tempo of the music picked up as the haircutters came to the conclusion of their performance. The models' hair designs were magnificent! They had created the ultimate looks for their ultimate clients on that day. The audience was standing and shouting in the aisles!

The Spoken Word

Finally, one of the artists put his hand up and gained the audience's immediate respect. This audience was not just haircutters, but colorists, perm specialists, receptionists, skin care people, cosmetic technicians, and nail technicians, and the artists had united them through their artistry!

There are certain principles that we on this platform believe to be the foundation for the successes of today and in the future. As during the haircuts, he systematically pointed them out. **Understanding and caring about who and what you are is the first step to successful hair designing. That caring also includes each and every member of your team. Being able to communicate this to your salon members as well as to your clients is crucial for your success.** *Looking as you have, and listening as intently as you are right now, is the third and final thought. We hope we have been an example to you today!*

The cosmetologist or barber-stylist who will be most successful will be the one who not only cuts well, but also works as a team player in the salon community. With a cooperative, helpful attitude, the pro will gain respect from other members of the work family. And the clientele will sense that respect.

THE SPECIALIST

The salon of the twenty-first century wouldn't be complete without the skills of the specialist. There are many special services offered in salons staffed with psy-cosmetologists. **The age of specialization is upon us.** No matter where we look, there is a specialist for every service imaginable. Whether we talk about advanced perm waving, design hair coloring, skin and cosmetic essentials, or specialists who perform manicures, nail wrapping or tipping, we are seeing growth in demand for the services.

These essentials have an influence on each and every team member, if only from the aspect of the specialist's ability to keep the staff looking fashion-conscious and trend oriented in all areas of beauty. This enhances the whole salon's value in the public eye.

From the clients' perspective, they seem to want the reassurance that each service performed for them is being given by a specialist. The ability of the chemical experts to influence clients on the enhancement of their hair through special services creates a natural bond between the chemical technicians and the rest of the staff. *The more services we render to one client,* one technician said, *the better our chances of maintaining the client for a longer period of time!*

Salon Make-Overs for a Professional Team Image

The chemical technician pointed out to us that we should attend one of their "salon make-over days." *This is where we spend the entire day designing make-overs for the staff. What an electrifying day of ideas, enthusiasm, and acknowledgement!* The specialist said, *We work very hard to further develop the rapport with our special staff members. We all get a chance to be pampered. It's a day when we as chemical technicians get a chance to explain the latest techniques in perming and hair coloring.*

The greatest enjoyment we get is our pride in being able to design the latest looks for each and every staff member. They appreciate our skills, and we enjoy theirs. We work with each other because we want our clients to really understand that we practice what we preach. We all design with the individual's needs in mind. Even though we're in the cosmetology profession, we still share some of the same fears clients feel when they come to the salon. **Our clients get encouragement from us to try something new when they see the results of our make-overs.** They say, "You really did get that new cut and color! How do you feel about the change?" We just smile, and they know!

After the designs are completed, and the chemical work is finished, we get the latest in skin tips and cosmetic applications. This gives us a chance to try new looks that we might not ordinarily try if it weren't for our specialist in skin and cosmetics encouraging us. Everyone is involved, including the receptionist with her total make-over, who just can't wait for tomorrow so she can show our clients her new look.

Getting Better Together

The specialist continued, *The change is so important to all of us because we want to keep improving ourselves. The cleansing technicians are running around telling us the latest in conditioners and treatments, and always a funny story is included about the shampoo hose getting loose and flying around the room! The haircutters are pressing the outer dimensions of their artistry so that we look number 1!*

Not enough can be said about the specialist who works with delicate chemicals to ensure formulas that present the finest in creative endeavors. Of course, the time, money, and learning that it takes to become a qualified specialist is hard to relate to. Making the thousands of formulations and reformulations is an art it itself.

The day would not be complete without everyone having his or her nails manicured or a special tipping applied. The total package of beauty that we give to each other is very special. We all are living examples of what we profess! What a confidence builder! Just imagine, it all started because one specialist felt it was important to have the whole salon doing these changes together.

We felt this exemplified the teamness of the twenty-first century salon. The receptionist, the cleansing technician, the hair designer, and the specialists are all an integral part of the salon team concept. The networking that we have been discussing is, and most often has to be, orchestrated by a special individual who walks a delicate tightrope among human feelings and emotions. Many times, the entire operation of an organization lies in the hands of one very special person. This person can be in one day a stylist, a receptionist, or a cleansing technician. We may know him or her as the twenty-first-century manager of the salon team.

THE MANAGER

The manager's role in the salon of the twenty-first century is laden with critical and numerous responsibilities. A manager is like an octopus reaching into many areas of the workplace at once, and is often required to make split-second decisions. For many salon managers, tasks and duties related directly to management comprise only a small part of their daily routine. Besides running the salon, 90 percent of all managers are also stylists, who spend a great portion of their days working behind the chair.

Naturally, to be totally successful as team leaders, managers must earn the respect of their entire staff and still provide management direction. Proficient managers have the ability to get the work load completed by involving the entire salon team in all aspects of salon development. Just as the owner needs a manager as a right-hand employee, the salon manager needs the staff to assist with the sometimes overwhelming salon tasks that must be accomplished.

Participative Management

In his best-selling book, *Theory Z,* William Ouchi points out that **the more workers are involved in the decision-making process, the more productive the overall organizations have been.** Ouchi, in describing many Japanese businesses, showed the productive result of workers rotating job positions to further develop themselves. Like a mother and father who care, oversee and protect, their managers insist that chances of long-term success will be enhanced by workers who grow and participate in all aspects of their specific businesses.

Some salon managers have the proverbial problem of staff members wanting to "play hooky." This is a result of boredom with repetitious work and the desire to escape. One hundred and eighty degrees to the opposite is the attitude of Japanese workers who put in long workdays, and actually look down on short work days as an indication that the employee is having a problem with his or her job.

Key Management Ingredients:
Attitude, Enthusiasm, Encouragement

Donna M. asserted that one of her most important responsibilities was to keep the attitude and the enthusiasm of the staff "perking along." Donna views each team member as a special individual and tries to understand his or her unique needs. In return, their performance is a reflection of her management ability.

Donna explains, *You get what you give, and I feel actions speak louder than words. I believe in leading by example for my team. People really want to work and get along together. Once in a while, the staff gets off track, and I gently help them get back on track. We all need that. Because of the vast amount of time we spend together in the salon, proper attitude and understanding of each other are critical! I try to represent all parties objectively. As the facilitator, and sometimes mediator, I must keep the channels of communication open with my staff. My staff knows I will speak up for them. After all, communication has always been a two-way street.*

Hiring for the Team

It sounds like Donna has a slick, well-running salon that truly represents the manager of the twenty-first century leading the salon team. The Human Revolution is showing us what is right with people. If we follow its direction, we can face the negative aspects more productively after a careful acknowledgement of what's right. As pointed out at a recent conference of managers and owners, their responsibilities often have the delicateness of walking a tightrope between the owner's and the staff's needs.

Often included in the hiring process of the salon, one manager stated, *When I'm hiring a new stylist, I consider the personality of each and every member of my staff, but especially their styling peers. I want my staff to know that our salon will grow from a new stylist addition, not slip backwards. Our staff is very conscious that a new team member will be interfacing with their clients, and we all want that interfacing to be positive!*

I often have informal conversations with my designers over a newly hired stylist, to take into consideration their perspectives. Involving them has been tremendously helpful in enlisting a positive attitude from them and gaining their acceptance of the new staff member. As a manager, I try to make the staff a part of the management decision whenever possible.

Starting Each Day the Right Way

Mary K. of Atlanta pointed out to us that one of her priorities as a manager was to be in the salon one hour earlier than the staff. She shared coffee and ideas with her receptionist to start off the day on a positive note. She went on to describe how their receptionist was the catalyst of the salon. This leader realized the demands that are put on the receptionist on a daily basis.

My whole staff needs my support from the beginning of the day. Whether the problems be big or small, they know they can depend on me. It's the start of the day that sets the tone for the rest of the salon's day.

"Put Your Ears on a Stick"

At a management program recently, author and lecturer Margaret Hamin and human relations consultant Christopher C. Reilly were developing the listening skills of a group of managers. Chris said, *You must put your ears on a stick!* The audience chuckled, as they honed in on the unusual statement. They opened up their ears for more explanation. **As a manager, listening can be one of your most valuable skills,** or "tools," *if you please.*

One of the participants spoke up, *Chris, I'd like to share an experience, because I think I understand what you're saying. I have tried to utilize my receptionist's talents with the staff to help me stay in tune with their needs. She has the innate knack of knowing what our staff is thinking! She really listens to what they say and never panics during crises. With the coolness of a sharpshooter 300 hundred yards away from the target, her piercing eyes tell me when she needs my attention, and somehow, we wind up in a conversation.*

Chris acknowledged, *Exactly! You're managing through other people's efforts and desire to assist. Bravo for your receptionist! The entire salon must feel comfortable. They have "ears" that will listen to them. You truly have a receptionist who has her "ears on a stick."*

No Good Morning, No Ears on a Stick

The well-tanned, rather muscular manager from San Diego commented, *Where I worked before, my manager was booked* every single day from when I came in until I left. I must admit, I was a little envious and wondered why he couldn't share some of these clients with me. I realized that this was small thinking, but that's how I felt. There was seldom a "good morning" or even an acknowledgement of me being there. I almost felt like I was imposing when I came near his domain! He was so busy, he had to have two styling chairs to keep up!

I remember other staff members and myself in the back having political salon caucuses about him. No one was brave enough to confront him, so we just gunnysacked our feelings. I was only in the beauty industry about a year when I started working there, and I thought I picked the wrong profession! First thing in the morning, without looking up, he would shout out orders to people in a machine-gun-like fashion. "You, get the towels and put them in the washer and fill the shampoo bottles." "You, call the distributor and tell him we're out of this or that and I want it today!" "You two will do Sue's clients today. Sue's sick again, per usual! Just split them up, I don't care how, just get them done!"

I look back now, and many days we looked like zombies on remote control. Our eyes deceived us and that clock on the wall showed no mercy. Once in a while, the manager would look up and say, "What's wrong with you?" How do you answer that one? I made a promise to myself that if I ever had the opportunity of managing a group of people, I would try not to practice any of the demoralizing, dehumanizing tactics I lived through. I'm happy to say I'm a successful team manager today, thanks to the cooperation of my staff.

What a Difference an Hour Can Make

One Denver, Colorado manager advised, *I start my day by not booking any clients for the first hour to hour and a half. I'm there before our staff arrives, to promote punctuality as a key to our overall success. I give all team members their morning space when they first come in, to let them adjust. A warm, friendly greeting meets my staff each and every day. Consistency shown to them produces consistency in them. Each individual has his or her own morning behavior patterns and I have learned my staff's. My objective, however, is to make contact over the first ninety minutes with each member. Many situations are cleared up because I'm there to make those decisions and have the time to do so.*

Just the other morning, a problem arose with our newest cleansing technician, who was confused about which shampoo to recommend to a client. Understanding her plight in being afraid to make a mistake, I again supported her. I also pointed out that if she was really undecided on what particular shampoo to use, some of her co-professionals would gladly help. I reassured her that all of us were also unsure when we started, and we realized what she was going through in this rather large transition. I encouraged her to put less pressure on herself, and reemphasized the fact that she has a manager to help! I thanked her for coming to me and letting me help, rather than keeping her uncertainties inside. I think she felt better.

Blending the New with the Old

The energy that new staff members bring to the team is like a transfusion of new ideas. Their ideas and talents are, to a great degree, going to be influenced by a manager's willingness to understand their needs and their willingness to perceive the manager's needs. Team managers are fortunate to have an opportunity to be a positive force in their young staff member's lives.

An astute, well-intentioned manager from Morristown, Pennsylvania, pointed out that a key to managerial success was to not play favorites. *For a period of two weeks, my perm and coloring specialists were not performing up to their normal capabilities. Their creativity and enthusiasm seemed to have dropped. They weren't sitting with me for morning coffee anymore. It seemed my space had become off limits to them.*

Thank God for other staff members who were really tuned in and have helped me out with my role as a manager. Our cosmetic artist came into my office and, like a gentle lioness, sat down and opened up. She said, "Bob, I think we have a problem here. The staff knows you have been busy lately with the three new salon members. I think they feel they have not been getting the time with you they need." I caught her piercing eyes, yet warmth of words. Her words ran through my mind and body. How easy it is to overlook the everyday performers who are the backbone of the salon! I just simply had been paying too much attention to our new members and not enough to the rest of the staff! I took care of the problem immediately!

From Losers to Winners

Another manager of a full-service salon related to us that he had several different specialists. *We have manicuring services, nail wrapping and nail tipping, skin care and cosmetic services,* along with the traditional cuts, perms, and conditioning. With this many people, it's essential to have team goals that we work towards together. I remember when I first took over as manager, I would have contests, and only the highest producer would win the prize. Everybody else was a loser! And I wondered why people wouldn't even try!

As a manager, I eventually realized that I was creating a losing, not a winning, team feeling between staff members. I still do believe in personal achievements, but now we set team goals where everybody shares. Everyone can win. If my staff members win, all the clients become the big winners!

Our staff appreciates that we don't put a big chart on the wall and expose their weaknesses. Rather, we work on modifying those areas together. People will grow faster and more positively when you do not humiliate them in front of their peers. **Take a person's pride away and you have a real problem with morale.**

As a manager, I know I have goals that must be met, and my staff does too. Each one is very aware of what his or her responsibilities are, and they try their hardest to fulfill those goals. They can't have their energies going toward disliking and feeling worthless. These are factors that cause low productivity and a sense of not caring. **Each staff member must know that his or her contribution is important to the salon,** or why will they put out the effort? The team manager must show them how their part of the contribution is essential to the growth of the salon team.

THE SALON OWNER

We have visited the worlds of the receptionist, the cleansing technician, the cosmetologist and barber-stylist, and the salon manager. We have explored the vital roles of each of these salon team players. But who is the ultimate overseer, father and mother, brother and sister, protector, provider, who dared to have the courage to trust the instincts that said, "GO FOR IT!"? These people are the Rocky Balboas and the Susan B. Anthonys of the world who wanted more and challenged themselves for it. They indeed had, as Dr. Lew pointed out, "the courage to be imperfect," to risk, and when they fell, they had the courage to get up and try again. These people are the original team salon players, the salon owners.

Leaders Are Not Always Loved

An owner of a salon tries to find ways to improve the salon's social and economic climate. Owners err frequently, but rebound to try again. There are many storms that have to be weathered to reign over a successful salon. Owners' dedication in taking on the responsibility of owning a salon says something for their Herculean character. As a clear path through the mountains shows trail packers the safeness of the journey, the owner who is a psy-cosmetologist is saying, "I accept the role of *leading* my salon by example." The path must be understandably clear. No one in the salon is more scrutinizing than the owner. Owners' decisions do not necessarily please each individual, but they decide what is best for the majority. The staff often looks to the salon owner as a team leader and team player, as the facilitator of more than just business affairs.

When They Fall, Pick Them Up

One owner suggested that the only way his staff would develop was by growing through solving problems themselves and having responsibilities to make decisions. *I was training a manager for my salon, Ron, who enjoyed people, assisted well, and generally was very helpful. I felt that Ron could develop into a fine decision maker. My responsibility was to show Ron that, as a new manager, he was going to have to encourage his staff to make some of their own decisions. I could see Ron was giving me only one-ear service.*

The time arrived, and Ron eagerly faced his new challenge as a manager. Ron had more responsibilities now. The staff members were asking him every little thing that had to be done. "Ron, what rods should I use? What do you think about this color? Ron, can you handle this problem on the phone?"

A few weeks later, Ron cornered me with a frenzied look on his face. "Please tell me what I'm doing wrong! I can't pay attention to my own clients. Everyone keeps interrupting me. I never thought it was going to be this difficult. You never seemed to have this many problems!"

I said to Ron as gently as I could, "What do you think the problem is?" Like a raging bull with fire spouting out of his nostrils, Ron bellowed, "If I knew what was wrong, do you think I would be asking you?" I attempted to calm down the visibly shaken manager.

He went on, "Everybody wants this, everybody wants that from me. I'm only one person, and I can't be everywhere all the time. This job is getting to me. Do these people think I'm God? I can't solve every problem!"

After listening, I helped him see how he had been his own worst enemy and that he should take some of the pressure off himself. I said, "I think you have the job wrong. You're not supposed to know all of the answers, but to help them find the answers. Let them work out most of the issues for themselves. But be there to support them! People grow through experiences and trying ideas, not by you or I telling them everything to do."

"Ron, I managed you for four years with seven other stylists, and I hope we grew because I had faith in the staff members' decision-making abilities. If you take on all the decisions, most people will let you do it."

The words were melting into Ron like the snow on a hot summer's day. "Thanks, Boss. I get the message loud and clear. Make them a part of the decision process. Trust that they are capable of participation."

I continued, "Ron, sometimes even a decision of which they are unsure gives them a chance to grow. If they fall, pick them up, and you will be just fine and so will they."

Ron has developed into an outstanding, delegating manager. As an owner, if I didn't have respect for my manager and my staff and belief in them, it would show right through like an x-ray showing a fragmented part of the body. That's how they would feel, and ultimately, no one would reach their goals on the team. It's not easy coaching from the sidelines, but champions are built by doing, not just telling. **Successful owners are team builders.**

Team Management

One of the most memorable experiences that I (Donald Scoleri) had was at a team management seminar in Cherry Hill, New Jersey. It was only 7:30 in the morning of a program that began at 10:00, and in walked two people who were dressed in a fashion that would make the most beautiful rainbow envious. As they walked down the center aisle, pride was evident in their bouncing steps, reminding one of the likes of Fred Astaire and Ginger Rogers. They introduced themselves and requested front-row seats, if possible. I obliged accordingly but was intrigued by their sunshiny facial expressions illuminating the area around them.

Bill introduced himself as the owner, and Rhonda represented herself as the receptionist/salon coordinator. *We know we're early. We've been driving since four o'clock this morning to get here!* This statement set me back! Rhonda, the reception-ist, spearheaded most of the conversation. Bill, the owner, was like a watchful observer, a proud father watching his offspring blossoming. As Rhonda shared their ideas on the financial responsibilities of a salon, you could see Bill mimicking through voiceless words, by movement of his lips. Rhonda pointed out that Bill had developed an ongoing education, advertising, and promotional budget for the salon. The entire staff was so in tune with how important these areas were for the total salon growth. They had the deepest respect for Bill, their owner.

Rhonda pointed out that not every salon has the guaranteed, built-in success plan that Bill had developed and had entrusted to Rhonda to carry out. She proudly shared, *I'm in charge of organizing all education events and advertising promotions. Bill oversees the entire operation, but we have the entire staff involved in the planning. Bill helped me organize myself and showed me how to get the information from the staff when I need it. Who would know more about what haircutters wanted to see and learn than the haircutters themselves? The chemical technicians knew what updatings were important to them. The specialist in the ever-changing world of skin care and cosmetics keeps us updated on the trends and fashions. When I first started working for Bill as his receptionist, I wanted to control everything. I didn't receive much cooperation. Bill understands us as people first and business employees secondly. That's why every staff member is willing to go the extra mile.*

The People Developing Owner

Bill has developed his staff, and Rhonda was proud to talk about their accomplishments with other people. As the respectful groups at the seminar brought their attention to Bill, he spoke. *As an owner like many of you, I have tried to put my life experiences to good use.* He gave these words of encouragement: *We have a normal responsibility to help our staff grow and mature. We often help mold a major part of their future. That's why they are an important part of the planning, because those plans involve them.*

The owner is like the five senses we often take for granted. Hearing what is not said, smelling the success that has not yet come while encouraging the team to reach and use all the assets within them. Touching them when human warmth is the only substance that will soothe their needs. Seeing what is there and forecasting like a crystal ball what is yet to come. Tasting the elegance of fruitful growth, that I as an owner had a major part in creating. I think my receptionist, Rhonda, is an example that I'm proud to call a salon staff professional. This owner was a true psy-cosmetologist who believed in building a salon team of involved people.

People and Education
Make the Difference

In September of 1983, we launched an exciting new concept in educational programming in New Orleans, Louisiana. The participants were an enthusiastic crowd of 325 professional cosmetologists, barber-stylists, and salon consultants. This was a dream come true, because the reality developed from the educational needs of salon people across America and Canada! The educational program was designed to have a permanent affect on the hearts and minds of the salon team members.

As we stood having an eye-opening cup of coffee, a gentleman, well-groomed and in vogue, approached us. Mr. Albert B. said, *Do you remember me? We met about three years ago.* Shaking my head no, I (Donald Scoleri) apologized that, *No, I do not.* Albert replied, *Well, I remember you and I'll quote you.* I felt the blood rushing to my face, hoping that I had not, in a foolish moment, spoken unjustly or delivered a poor message.

Once you said that education had changed your life, and I want to thank you, because education has changed my business life and also my personal life. Do you remember how you described your feelings that you were afraid to raise prices, because you knew you weren't doing anything different? But, your real internal fear was of losing clients and revenue? I acknowledged. *Or when you shared how you lost your first staff because of no guidance and direction, because you just didn't have the educational background?*

His words struck with accuracy, giving me a sense of déjà vu. *But most of all, how education had broadened the scope of your world, and that one of your vital organs, your family, "paid the price" for your unhappiness. You explained how they could be adjusted and put into perspective.* Anxiously, I answered, *Yes, yes! I remember so well all those experiences!*

I could not let you go on stage today without letting you know that three years ago I had a rather small staff and some of those same fears. With his chest expanding like King Kong, he produced a smile, warmth, and calmness that brought immediate tranquility to me.

Don, I'm proud to tell you that the first two rows are my staff members! In proud acknowledgement, he pointed to his well-groomed, professional-looking staff. *You and your wife must feel great about your accomplishments,* I said. *Yes, we're proud of what we, not I, have accomplished.*

A salon owner can be like a still lake on a warm summer's night. With high technology and well-developed people communication, our lake seems to have movement and momentum it never had before. Thanks Don. As we walked away, Lew and I looked at each other and heaved a sigh of relief!

It's Lonely at the Top

One of the most rewarding stories we can share with you is about a salon owner from Canada who told us that her business had grown so quickly, she felt she did not have control of the salon, and that changes were needed. Having thirteen employees is no easy thing. She felt she had good people and wanted to make a brighter future for everyone. One thing she felt she had developed was a salon relationship with the clientele bordering on the spectacular. Her keenness to make each and every client feel that he or she was "the one and only" made this her foremost goal. This had spread through most of the staff. But change often doesn't. Confrontation occurred, and three of her top' stylists gave her an ultimatum. There was an uneasiness within the salon and among the clients. To her shock, a few of the clients came to her and said that a few of her stylists were thinking of leaving, and they felt uncomfortable. This process continued for about two weeks.

I Believe in Me and You

Her response was a declaration of pride and understanding not many owners might even want to choose as an alternative. She told each client, *You know how I have established our salon. I believe all our stylists do quality design work and that we have first and foremost always put you as our number one priority. If some of my stylists leave, we will go on, and I want you to know whatever decision you make now or in the future, our salon will always be open to you.*

She said many of the clients were a little surprised at her nonaggressive attitude. *My attitude is to do what is best for my existing clientele. Friction and unhappiness are not attributes to look up to.*

I finally talked to my staff members one at a time and explained that I understood and respected their feelings and opinions. They had helped the salon grow. As the owner, I had to make some lonely business decisions after getting all the input from them. They had heard my decisions. I told them, "I care for you. I believe we can have a bright future together. The decision is yours!"

We later received a call from this young lady. Final count, not one stylist lost, business growing beautifully. Her commitment to herself, her staff, and her clients made for a happy ending.

The positive interaction of receptionist, cleansing technician, stylist, specialist, manager, and owner is a necessary ingredient for the successful twenty-first-century salon.

HIGHLIGHTS FROM CHAPTER 3

In Chapter 3 we uncovered the importance of the effects of social change on an entire profession, from the individualistic thinking of the 1950s and 1960s to the blossoming from "me thinking" to "we thinking" salon employees. A major emphasis of Chapter 3 was on how **the new psy-cosmetologist realizes, with uncanny accuracy, the inescapable need for all employees to work as a team.**

1. The changing size of salons of the 1950s and 1960s when stylists functioned as individuals has been replaced in the 1980s by the base of salon employees, which in some cases has quadrupled in size, creating a need for effective communication and teamwork.

2. Social changes created the need for salon professionals to develop people skills, to promote harmony and unity in the salons and barber-styling establishments.

3. Individual attitudes were replaced by task-oriented, team attitudes, which benefitted everyone, especially the clients.

4. Dedicated team players now show they are in tune with society's needs by developing an incredibly warm and safe environment for clients, and by reaching out to help the community.

Chapter 3 focused on each salon employee and showed how each member of the team has a positive affect on every other team member, which ultimately affects clients.

- **The Receptionist:** stage setter, image maker, and public relations ambassador.

- **The Cleansing Technician:** dedicated to the comfort of the client, and a critically important person in the overall success of the entire salon. The cleansing technician is a person who gives a therapeutic massage one moment and answers the phone the next. The interaction of these functions is totally essential.

- **The Cosmetologist or Barber-Stylist:** front-liner who finds the delicate and important balance between technical and communicative skills, knowing he or she has the power to transform people with his or her skills. The cosmetologist's or barber-stylist's effective communication creates a magical atmosphere that is totally satisfying.

- **The Specialist:** specializes in a specific area of endeavor and excels at the task. Has the unique ability to put the finishing touches to the artistic design.

- **The Manager:** dedicated team player who, like an octopus, reaches into every area of the salon and finds the magic to make everyone want to work as a team. The manager's role changes dramatically on any given day, often requiring him or her to act as a buffering force to maintain a well-balanced, team-oriented salon.

- **The Salon Owner:** the special individual who is the ultimate overseer, often the father and mother, brother and sister, protector, provider, and foundation of the salon. He or she took the risk to "go for it" and realizes the importance of developing team players for a successful future. Often not loved for his or her decisions, but respected for the ability to make decisions, the manager's foresight has made the difference in creating incredible, positive changes that have blessed our profession.

We have addressed in Chapter 1 the special relationship between the psy-cosmetologist and the client. Chapter 2 looked at the unique qualities of the new psy-cosmetologist. Chapter 3 represented the benefits of team players. Chapter 4 projects and clarifies the trends and the impact these trends will have on clients, highlighting the new psy-cosmetologist as a human relations specialist.

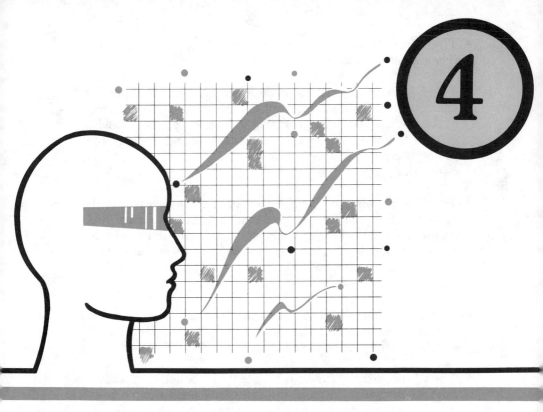

The New Psy-Cosmetology: A Glance At The Trends

TREND 1: THE NEW PSY-COSMETOLOGIST: A HUMAN RELATIONS SPECIALIST

As we discussed in Chapters 1 and 2, there will be an increasing emphasis on the quality of the relationship between the psy-cosmetologist and the client. Although many other factors will reshape the profession, the human relations specialist with an understanding of how to handle human encounters will continually spiral in importance.

Almost every successful business strives for optimum client awareness. This closeness is exemplified in the actions of the new psy-cosmetologist. **The sensitive stylist with positive attitude, outward confidence, and desire to cooperate with other team members has the edge.**

When considering that human relationships are the cornerstone to self-development, and that the clients' hair is one of the most important factors of their physical and emotional well-being, you begin to realize the special confidence clients must have in their stylists. Obviously, **clients will have more trust in stylists who have taken the time to develop their human relations skills.** This is the human relations specialist that we are seeing in increasing numbers in the professions of cosmetology and barber-styling.

Who Are These Human Relations Specialists?

The human relations specialists are the most talented, sensitive individuals currently in the profession. They have been developing their human relations and technical skills in almost every corner of our country, from the City of Brotherly Love, Philadelphia, Pennsylvania, to the car capital of Detroit, Michigan, to the snow-covered fields of Minnesota; in the milk-fed cattle lands of Iowa, Kansas, and Nebraska; and near the crashing rapids of the Grand Canyon. They earn the recognition of being psy-cosmetologists from their peers and society alike, because they personify excellence in human relations and caring. You will find them conducting formal and informal sessions in their own towns, helping fellow professionals to get in tune.

Slowly, but inevitably, cosmetology and barber-styling schools are incorporating human relations training into their fine technical programs to round out their students. As a psychologist, I (Lew Losoncy) have worked in schools in over a dozen states and have observed cosmetology schools in Iowa City and New Orleans with psychologists on staff. There are others.

Successful Salons House
Human Relations Specialists

We have found that successful salons are obsessed with sensitivity to the client, regardless of staff size. **Top notch salons take the time to develop specific strategies to give their valued clients quality service and a positive appearance.** Among the thousands of examples of client sympathy we have observed, five primary elements seem to be common to the most successful salons. These common ingredients are creating psychological safety, identifying the positive aspects of people, supporting co-professionals in the clients' eyes, gaining client confidence through consulting, and seeking feedback on technical services and personal treatments.

Creating Psychological Safety for Clientele

Psy-cosmetologists recognize that clients develop their attitudes about salons (like, dislike; warm, cold; friendly, unfriendly; relaxed, tense) **immediately upon entering the reception area.** Surveys indicate that their emotional mood develops seconds after first-time clients enter the "strange home." The decision to come back to the salon is often made even before the first technical application is performed.

Psychological safety is facilitated by a warm smile and a friendly greeting. This is fulfilled through an introduction by the salon professional, an inquiry into the person's name. Only after psychological climate is established is the issue of technical services addressed.

Identifying Positive Aspects of People

The psy-cosmetologists we observed seem to get the relationship off on a positive note by identifying positive

101

features about their clients. This could include appearance; hair, skin, or nail assets; personality traits; and clothing. They maintain this positive feeling by continually highlighting the person's plus points and by using a positive vocabulary. (See Chapter 2 on the REACH Concept.)

Supporting Co-Professionals

The psy-cosmetologist shares outstanding assets about other members of the staff that will give the client a feeling of confidence in all staff members. A secondary benefit of one stylist's complimenting another is that it shows the client that the salon atmosphere is filled with warmth and caring, not jealousies, and that more than one stylist is capable of taking care of his or her needs.

Gaining Clients' Confidence

The psy-cosmetologist frequently provides initial consultations that gain the clients' confidence from both a technical and a human relations standpoint. In some salons, this is done using the REACH Client Asset Card (see Chapter 2). Knowing the powers of first impressions, the psy-cosmetologist realizes that this consultation can dramatically increase client retention rates. At this consultation, many psy-cosmetologists offer a personal money-back guarantee on all services and products. This statement of confidence offers an all-win situation to the client and exemplifies good human relations at its finest.

Seeking Feedback

Psy-cosmetologists' appointments are not completed until they understand clients' perceptions of the salon experience, from both a technical and a personal perspective. **One of the most frequent mistakes salons make is to send clients off without finding out what their feelings were about the salon experience.** Human relations oriented salons nip dissatisfaction in the bud by getting feedback and making necessary changes. Secure professionals see feedback as the ultimate opportunity for growth.

TREND 2. SENSITIVITY TO
HIGH-TECH/HIGH TOUCH

Trend 1 addressed the salon environment from a human perspective, that is, the stylists' attitudes and behaviors and how they affect the clientele. No less important is a second trend that we observed, which is the development of the right physical atmosphere in salons. This is the obvious reason professional salons are putting a greater accent on the physical and psychological image the salon environment projects. In this high-tech world, it is necessary for salons to offer the surroundings that are most sensitive to their targeted markets.

Balancing High-Tech with High-Touch

The physical and psychological environment of salons staffed by psy-cosmetologists reflects the high-tech/high-touch era in which we are living. This reflection illuminates through the personnel and ultimately shines on the clients. High technology, without touch, is sterile; high touch without technology is antique. In the Human Revolution, the only long-term approach to salon growth is to bring the technical and human aspects together in balance.

If you will allow us some poetic license, we would like to take you on an imaginary visit to experience a sample of a high-tech/high-touch oriented salon of the future. On your experimental visit, keep your mind close to the high-technical components of this salon, and keep your heart and five senses in tune with the high-touch aspects of this imaginary salon. If both your mind and heart are ready, let's begin our visit.

As you stand outside the salon, your mind and senses already start to develop an imaginary picture of what you are about to experience. You are encouraged by its inviting appeal, which generates a theme of professionalism coupled with warmth. You like it, and somehow or other, you trust it. You enter.

The Central Control Center

After a warm, cheerful greeting and a handshake from the unpretentious receptionist, you are encouraged to find a seat. As you search the reception area, you find yourself enticed to sit in a comfortable looking chair. Attached earphone sets are available for your pleasure. You notice several monitor screens above the receptionist's desk and a code sequencer on the arm of each lounge chair. In front of you is an electric salon menu that runs automatically, with a pause sequence between each printout describing all the special services available to you and their estimated costs. You are intrigued to find that approximate times are suggested for all the services.

The receptionist is sensitive to your curiosity and encourages you to explore further. All those monitors excite you and you want to know what's behind each one. You select monitor one, and up flashes cartoons for the kids and a variety of games for their amusement. You wish you could share this experience with that special little one you know. Next comes the teen's monitors with the latest in clothing and hair fashions worn by their musical and screen idols. The next monitor shows you special techniques in perm waving and hair coloring, and the next a variety of haircut designs.

Your excitement grows as you accelerate your speed to get to the treasure behind the next compelling monitor. This monitor is discussing how to take care of your hair, skin, and nails by realizing all of their assets, not just the liabilities. The intriguing word *REACH* comes on your monitor. Then the computer spells out REACH for you: *R*elating through *E*mphasizing the *A*ssets in the *C*lient's *H*air. Please ask your stylist for further information.

The final two monitors attract your interest the most because they are designated "special, first-time visit information." The orchestrated video meticulously waltzes you through each step of your salon visit, and you can feel the anxiety slowly leaving your body. You are enthralled that every minute detail has been clearly defined for your personal gratification. Your senses tell you that this is a far cry from a few years ago, when you last visited a design parlor.

Thank You for Noticing Me!

You search around the receptionist area, and you cannot help but notice the sparkling, multi-colored, well-lighted display areas. The displays of professional products seem to wrap endlessly around the spacious room, so as to be noticed from any sitting or standing position. You marvel at the rotating glass shelving that comes out of the wall, hesitates a few seconds, and then disappears! Immediately, new merchandise appears, enticing you to walk over and get more acquainted.

You reach out to pick up a specialized asset-oriented shampoo and are startled beyond belief by a voice that says, *Thank you for noticing me! My name is I Care For You Shampoo. I come in these exotic fragrances. Please open me up and smell me. Thank you for caring about me and your hair. For further assistance, just ask any of our qualified staff consultants or the receptionist standing behind you.* You turn around, and there she is! You're startled until she explains that the glass is sensitized, and when a client touches a product, special lights around the salon go on. Someone from the staff becomes available for assistance.

The high-tech talking retail rack and the human service are incredible! You had dreamed about it, but now you are finally experiencing it! You are so impressed with the convenience of the establishment. As you stand there by the displays, a gentle breeze passes you. You realize no particles of dust will ever settle here because of the salon's sensitivity to cleanliness. It occurs to you that, if they are that sensitive to having a clean display, they will be ultra-sensitive with you, a person. You feel important! Your intrigue grows as you enter the second phase of your cosmetic appointment. Before you can say "What's next?" the receptionist hands you your REACH Client Asset Computer Card.

A Refreshing Experience

By the time the cleansing technician escorts you to the cleansing area, you know that a pleasant experience is at hand. Your computer-printed Client Asset Card accompanies you to the cleansing technician's lounge. You recline into a body-shaped chair, which engulfs you with the soft gentleness of a warm spring day. The cleansing technician's skilled and caring touch, coupled with the technologically controlled water temperature and pressure, creates within you a feeling of relaxation.

High-Tech/High-Touch Styling

You now enter the psy-cosmetologist's styling area, where you are greeted by a sea of friendly faces. The warm feeling of the styling area is inviting, and the warmth overwhelms you. Although the room has great openness, the architectural design makes you feel you have your own private area.

High-Tech/High-Touch at its Peak

Your eyes scan the styling area in disbelief. At each station there are TV monitors being used by the psy-cosmetologists for their individual audiences. The dyads seem to be entranced, deep in their conversations and oblivious to the world around them.

Your psy-cosmetologist tells you that before any service will be performed, all your questions will be answered so that you can be comfortable with your decision. You are presently being video taped, informed that all of your likes and dislikes will be fed into the computer. Your psy-cosmetologist will enter his or her recommendations, and composites of hair designs will be presented to you. You are also exposed to a variety of fashion waves and hair coloring designs that will best suit you and your lifestyle. Next, an array of cosmetic colors best suited to your natural coloring appears on the screen. To finalize a dream come true, the monitor flashes wardrobes of casual, midday, and evening apparel. All of this before even a lock of hair has been removed. You, with the assistance of your psy-cosmetologist, make your choice. For the first time in your life you feel truly confident in your judgment.

More to Come

As the psy-cosmetologist gently tilts your head forward, a snake-like chin rest comes up from the side of the styling chair. You find your chin gently resting in the pouch-like apparatus. Your only thought is, "What can be next?" The designing of the nape of your neck is soon completed. Your head is tilted from side to side. It does not hang out in limbo, but rests again in the soft pouch, while the designer cuts the opposite side of the design.

As the design is completed, your feeling of contentment runs over. The smile that covers your entire face is gratification enough to the psy-cosmetologist. As a soft breeze-like stream comes from the ceiling, your styling chair turns ever so slowly, to cleanse any minute particles of hair from your face and neck. To your astonishment, your completed hair design appears on all the other psy-cosmetologists' computers and draws smiles from designers and clients alike that make you feel special. Your monitor shows every aspect of your hair design. You just feel so good, words can't express your inner feelings!

The psy-cosmetologist thanks you and offers the services of the specialist in cosmetics to enhance your striking features. Like

Picasso with a brush, the cosmetic specialist quickly and delicately completes the *Mona Lisa* of your life—you! You are escorted to the central control center, where the smiling and acknowledging receptionist agrees with your choice of design. The overwhelming sentiment that runs through your body is something that you will never forget and anticipate experiencing again.

The Final Step

As a result of your hair analysis from the REACH Client Asset Card and the recommendation from your psy-cosmetologist, the receptionist has filled out your personalized home hair care enhancement regime. Every step has been taken care of for you, even to the plastic laminated code enhancement chart for your shower, to make each step successful and not wasteful.

You are assured that any information you may need has been put into your educational take-home kit. There is a special list of numbers you can dial to receive direct information on any other services you might wish to receive. You are guaranteed to receive the salon newsletter, with updates on hair, skin, and nail information and any special promotions that might be offered. You are thanked by a team of people who have combined the best of technology and touch to build an environment for you. You know you have ascended into the twenty-first-century salon of tomorrow . . . or is it really today?

Your imaginary salon visit is over . . . or is it? No, increasingly salons and barber-styling establishments have moved toward creating an environment with high technology and high touch to give you, the client in the Human Revolution, a choice. Most of the twenty-first-century ideas you have just experienced already exist in some forms.

TREND 3. SENSITIVITY TO CLIENTS' CHANGING NEEDS

Many salons have become quality-service oriented. That is, in addition to providing haircutting, perming, and coloring services, many salons offer such other services as skin care, manicuring, pedicuring, body wrapping, and massage. They are directly meeting the comprehensive changing needs of the quality-service oriented client as well. Quality of service rendered and the amount of money spent will have a direct effect on salon growth. **The quality client in the Human Revolution wants consistency of performance and will respond by supporting those who give it.** That is the position of the new psy-cosmetologist who uses knowledge to its fullest dimension to satisfy the client!

Multi-Optional Clients

It is very obvious to us that clients have become aware of the many options available to them. They want and demand freedom of choice. The standardized looks that clients have worn for years are less popular. Clients express an ever-increasing desire to change their looks on a much more frequent basis. From constant cosmetic designer changes to variety of apparel, no one element controls their fantasies for too long. They are not bashful in their approaches to life. If they want something, they will seek out those who can provide it. Price is not a barrier in most cases.

Clients' Spending Habits

The most lucid fact that has captured our imagination is the clients' acceptance of spending inordinate amounts of money on health, hygiene, and hair care. For years, salons have limited clients' options. **Today's clients have proven in the marketplace that when multi-option purchase alternatives are available, their buying power in some cases has doubled.**

In the January 6, 1984 issue of *U.S.A. TODAY*, Sears, Penney's and other major retail stores dramatically pointed out that over 60 percent of all Christmas sales for 1983 were credit oriented. These corporations have had to adapt to consumers' needs. They couldn't be competitive with just cash, checks, and their own credit cards. The multi-optional society forced the change, and at the end of 1983, these corporations found that over 50 percent of their total sales were credit. Simply put by one executive, "Credit is essential to good business today and in the future."

Today's consumers have a fast-paced style, and an almost radical approach to protecting their "fun time." They frequent salons less often, but purchase service in multi-units rather than one service at a time. A quality salon with major services will provide clients with the options necessary to create large-volume service and retail advancements.

Plastic Money

It is increasingly obvious that progressive salons give clients the option of purchasing services and retail merchandise not only with cash, but also with checks, credit cards, and some with their own private credit system.
Clients today spend ready cash almost as fast as they accumulate it! With the increase in cost of services and products, the fact is that clients are spending much more per visit. These options are necessary; credit is here to stay! It is the accepted way for clients to purchase today. The profession is just moving along with other professions, and its growth is unlimited, unless its practitioners themselves limit it! The client has clearly put the message out to all businesses, "Don't limit my buying power!" And we will respond.

Quality-service salons project that over the next decade the service ticket could triple in size, which puts even more pressure on the industry to adapt on the salon level to the quality service that clients want. The logical conclusion is to allow clients to choose how they want to purchase services and products.

The Age of Information and Service

The projections clearly indicate that a library of information and educational materials is necessary in the salon for the ever-inquisitive client. Quality-service clients are living in what John Naisbitt called the "New Information Age" in *Megatrends*. Clients have come to expect immediate information from professionals in all areas. Mass media has trained clients to expect instantaneous data. Clients look to cosmetologists as logical authorities on hair, skin, and nails. They are the doctors when it comes to cosmetic enhancement. With all the forms of information available, psy-cosmetologists can and do keep their clients totally abreast of fashions and trends to keep them in style.

Quality and Service are Here to Stay

It is important to note that, with the changing times, quality-service clients are no longer awed by one-service specialty salons. Clients have more self-trust and are more secure about decision-making when it comes to their hair, skin and nails. It's not just status that makes clients choose their salons, nor just one special service, but the quality-service image. Clients are keenly aware that no longer are there only a few excellent haircutting establishments, but thousands. The importance hasn't worn off, but the mystique of the haircut has.

The Lost Face

I'm the customer who comes into the clothing store and waits patiently for a salesperson to come!

I'm the customer who comes in to have one tire changed, and you try to pressure me to buy four new ones!

I am the customer who asked nicely for rare meat, and you made excuses.

I'm the customer whose warranty is still valid, and you give me all sorts of grief!

I'm the customer who doesn't say I am very unhappy with my hair, but you noticed and never did anything about it!

You think I am afraid and cowardly, or not assertive enough, and maybe you are right!

But I am also someone else that you try to remember, but can't.

I am the lost face, who just goes elsewhere to find contentment and service, without asking for it!

Truly, aren't we all that customer?

The psy-cosmetologist desires to meet the changing needs of clientele.

TREND 4. THE INVOLVEMENT OF COMPUTERIZATION

Small businesses can no longer manually perform all the business functions needed to keep them cost effective. The high tech of computerization gives salons the freedom to spend quality time in all other priority areas of their businesses. The emphasis on putting out a multitude of mini brushfires on a daily basis is over! Management's major responsibility is to lead its people to ongoing productivity and growth. With the capabilities of computerization, the salon of the future will have at its fingertips reports and listings in every crucial area of business. **Increasing productivity through computerization is in reality protecting a business investment and providing greater security for the future.**

A People Saver

When we review the awesome responsibilities of salon owners and staff alike, it is truly mind boggling! Besides working behind their styling chairs, their duties include dealing with people, money, advertising, hiring, ordering, problem solving, goodwill ambassadoring, and receptioning. Shall we go on? There are many areas that are delegated to staff members, such as manually controlling inventory, ordering supplies, and helping with direct mail advertising.

Let's explore just a few ways in which computerization can dramatically reduce the time and expense of overall business operation. Just as the experiences at Kitty Hawk changed the world of aviation, so has the role of computerization been propelled to higher altitudes in the salon. Time, patience, and perseverance will make the adjustment to computerization palatable.

Focusing on the big picture, **computers are automated assistants that help manage the salon, allowing owners and managers the flexibility to work in the areas that need immediate personal attention.** The computer captures the information necessary to focus attention into specific areas. The essence is that black and white doesn't lie. The facts are there faster and are more precise than those done by manual computation. The keys to more productivity are to have at hand stylist and client data which are produced on a daily basis. Yes, everything moves faster and at the same time more factually. As a result, issues can be dealt with more quickly and crises can be averted.

Imagine the tremendous pressure that comes off the salon personnel's shoulders when they enjoy these benefits of the computer. Salons are realizing they can grow with computerization if they give it a chance. The computer can do this and more:

COMPUTER ANALYSIS SYSTEM

- Daily Cash Reports
- Transactional Listings
- Client Information Analysis
- Client Record Cards
- Client Consultation Forms
- Client Master Listings
- Client Mailing Labeling
- Salon Performance Analysis
- Salon Review Analysis
- Salon Advertising Analysis
- Psy-Cosmetologist Weekly/Monthly Quality Report
- Payroll System
- General Ledger

- Accounts Payable
- Inventory Management System
- Inventory Master System
- Inventory Shortage System
- Inventory Usage System
- Inventory Cost System
- Inventory Receipts System

The twentieth century has produced the need for computer-ization. It will not disappear! **The future growth of the salon profession and all other professions depends on how quickly they adapt to finding that "new balance" so desparately needed between computerization (high tech) and high touch.**

TREND 5. EMPHASIS ON PERSONAL STANDARDS

A great shift has taken place in the professional and personal standards of the real pros in the industry. We observed with fascination the fact that **new psy-cosmetologists seem to have a strong code of professional ethics. They live by codes of self-reliance, personal responsibility, and social interest.** This unwritten code comes from within, much like the intuitional behavior of birds who migrate rhythmically with the changing seasons. They need not be told it's winter and time to go south. The new psy-cosmetologists know where to be and when to be there.

In their inner directiveness, psy-cosmetologists optimistically believe that they can remake the world, or at least those parts of the world that don't fit in with their common sense. Interestingly, their behaviors are similar to the self-trust that Maslow saw as present in self-actualized people. Maslow described healthy human beings, or advanced scouts for the human race, as being those who weren't afraid to take charge of their lives.

These self-actualized or new psy-cosmetologists are standing out, being felt, and being heard in every city and neighborhood in the world. They have taken a photograph of themselves and their industry and are redesigning the picture to make it more consistent with their personal standards, which are way beyond any standards that an external force could exert.

That's why new psy-cosmetologists are successful. They need not be told how to treat a customer, because they inherently know that **the way you treat other people reflects what you think of yourself.** They need not be told to cooperate, because they see themselves living in a world of equals.

One psy-cosmetologist manager who was unaware she belonged to this category said, My image has an important effect on the perception of the client towards me, and it is this, the client's perception, that ultimately determines how successful I will be. She, like many other psy-cosmetologists we observed, had an internal set of standards that guaranteed external success.

TREND 6. CHANGING SCOPE OF SALON HOURS

One of the major facts that the salon must resolve is the dramatic need for expanded salon hours or an adjustment of them. This issue of salon business hours will have an escalating affect on salon profitability. This naturally forces an extra demand on salon personnel because of the small structure of the average salon. Yet the facts are there; a changing society demands changing hours. **The once-standard salon hours are being challenged because of tremendous growth in the work force and the enormous need for clients to protect their social time.**

Women in the Work Force

It is projected that by the mid 1990s approximately 70 percent to 75 percent of all the women in America over the age of seventeen will be joining the massive work force, either on a full-time or part-time basis. This projection alone has forced professionals to rethink how salons can best service their clients. Time is a precious commodity to most clients, but especially to working clients.

Clients today do not perceive that they have a "special day" for a haircut or whatever services they want rendered. Due to precision cuts and minimum maintenance, a client can get a haircut at 10:00 at night as well as 10:00 in the morning. An evening or Sunday cut is acceptable social behavior. All other businesses, such as banks, drugstores, food stores, clothing stores, and gas stations, have realized that clients will shop or buy twenty-four hours a day when given the option.

Visit Less, Spend More

Clients want and make their schedules bend to their social needs. Clients look for businesses that respond to their needs. They are receiving multi-services at quality service salons because this will protect some of their time. This naturally will increase the spending of each client per visit. The down side for the industry is that **between 1985 and 1995, clients will visit salons approximately five or six rather than seven to ten times per year, but more clients than ever will go to salons, and they will spend more money.**

The Time Shift is Already Occurring

Our surveys show that most salons are booked to capacity from 4 o'clock on, no matter which evening they are open. Evening hours are the most understandable because of the enormous work force that is traditionally unavailable for morning and early afternoon appointments. **We project three major changes occurring in salon time schedules:**

1. **Salons will be open five to six nights a week, as they see the clientele migrate more to evening hours.**

2. **Salons will be open seven days a week for ever-moving clients.**

3. **Eventually salons will have 8-hour days, sharing shifts and rotating staff to fulfill clients' needs.**

We see the far-reaching objective will be that some salons will remain open 24 hours a day! If you doubt that, consider the fact that Las Vegas and many other resort and convention cities are already considering the possibility. The trend is also to eliminate standing appointments so consumers on the move can stop in anytime they see that "open" sign!

TREND 7. TELECOMMUNICATION TO BUILD CLIENTELE

The telephone is one of the most used technologies of all time, and yet one of the tools least utilized by the salon. Telephone communication or "tele-selling" is one of the major steps forward in developing a more cost-effective business. Progressive psy-cosmetologists realize and understand that we live in an information age, and people in society desperately want their information as soon as they can receive it. The direction is clear. Salons can't sit back and wait for clients to call them. **Salons are a service and information business, and telecommunication will be one of the most powerful tools to help develop the concept of "closeness to the client."**

Staying in Touch

When a client doesn't show up for an appointment, what do some salons do? Many get angry that the client didn't have the courtesy to call and cancel. Many business-sensitive salons take the responsibility of calling clients the day before to confirm their appointments. That's telecommunication in the purest sense— taking the action to show clients that salon people care!

When we introduced telecommunication to southern California salon owners, we encouraged them to go through their records for a year and see the tremendous dollars lost by the number of "no-shows," not to mention the unhappy stylists who were stood up and missed other potential bookings. **Telecommunication is quickly becoming the major means to stay in touch with salon clientele.**

Many salons are now canvassing their local telephone directories, realizing that each name in there is a potential client. Telecommunication will create new client bases through telephone canvassing. Telecommunication will eventually become a major part of salon advertising.

Market Expansion and Increased Profitability

1. **Telecommunication creates more of a demand for the the salon and its services by continually going after a new clientele base.**

2. **Telecommunication creates quicker service return of clients for more service and retail dollars.**

3. **Telecommunication reduces the overall down time of salons by decreasing no-shows.**

4. **Telecommunication creates a way of presenting salon benefits to clients.**

5. Telecommunication creates improved communication with clients.

6. Telecommunication creates a way of updating salon promotions that are of special interest to clientele.

7. Telecommunication creates a way of surveying the client base, both new and prospective.

8. Telecommunication creates an ongoing relationship with salon clients from visit to visit.

Considering all the indications that clients' visits to salons are decreasing on a per-year basis, clients are spending more per visit. It is then essential to stay in touch as much as possible with them. The psy-cosmetologist is moving quickly to utilize tele-communications.

TREND 8. EXPANDING POTENTIAL THROUGH EDUCATION

Ongoing education has been and will continue to be the cornerstone of the professional salon industry's growth. Psy-cosmetologists are fully aware that knowledge is everything and that unless they reach out for more education they remain the same. Clients are sensitive to seeing plaques and degrees at the stylists' stations. They know who went to the educational program on Monday and who didn't. Just as they want their doctors and dentists to continue their education, so they pride themselves on selecting hair "doctors" who crave education. Clients benefit from the expanded options that their stylists' education provides.

Manufacturers as Educators

Manufacturers have been leaders in the technical development and communicative growth of the profession. Utilizing their research and development laboratories, manufacturers add credibility to the salon in the clients' eyes by their constant breakthroughs in hair, skin and nail technology. Salons are depending on continued updatings to keep consumers in tune with those advances.

The thousands of educational programs that are held yearly by manufacturers are a source of growth for salons

of the future. Many manufacturers have entered the high-tech world of video. Video is quickly becoming a greater part of ongoing salon training.

Progressive manufacturers are sponsoring their own technicians and have brought education right to the salons' doorsteps! Whether it will be a multi-media presentation with the flash of Las Vegas or a small in-salon class, manufacturers are being asked on an ever-increasing basis to help lead the educational future of the professional salon industry.

Distributors as Educators

One of the major leaders in education has been the quality-service distributor of beauty and barber products. **No one entity is more closely associated with the salon level than the progressive distributorship with its tentacles of salespeople that touch almost every salon.** They feel and sense the pulse of needs on a daily basis, and they can react to these needs faster than anyone else.

Distributors are dramatically aware of the enormous role they are playing in the salon's success. Some have diversified their resources to put education in the forefront of the services they render. Some quality-service distributors have even built and organized their own educational centers where every form of educational class can be presented to fill the psy-cosmetologist's appetite for learning. Every conceivable class that pertains to hair, skin, and nails is available.

Futuristic distributors, realizing that technical skills need a balance of strong management training and communication skills, are making these forms of education a priority. Manufacturers, distributors, and salons know the importance of education and are utilizing it.

TREND 9. SOUND MANAGEMENT PRACTICES

The success of any business depends upon how it utilizes four natural resources: people, money, time, and facility. The salon business is leaving its embryonic stage of management and is maturing into a more sophisticated approach to management.

Addressing the priorities, rather than sporadically jumping from issue to issue, the salon becomes more cost effective and productive. The projections are clear: freewheeling, unorganized salons will not withstand the accelerated pace of change necessary to nourish their futures. **Finding a balance between technical aspects and managerial skills is crucial to running a successful business.** Increasingly, salon owners and managers are shifting priorities from cutting hair to overseeing business. To reach their business potential, managers must put more time into developing the four resources they have to work with.

Plan, Organize, Implement, Review

Twenty-first-century salons are not guessing at their futures. They're not hoping that profits are going to increase. They are planning in order to make things happen! Owners, managers, and stylists alike know that **planning, organizing, implementing, and reviewing are the ways to successful financial futures.** The progressive, futuristic leaders are directing their plans and are convinced of their merits. Most importantly, they see that true management needs constant monitoring and adjustment to fulfill the desired plans.

People Planning

It is our observation, agreed with by many owners, managers, and staff, that **people are the most important resource in the salon.** Because the salon profession is service intensive, service cannot reach its pinnacle without the salon developing its people. When a salon makes a firm commitment to developing people and realizes that in the end *people make the difference,* it moves forward.

The Differential Competitive Advantage

These salons achieve the differential competitive advantage that lecturer and author Christopher C. Reilly describes. Reilly, author of *Salon Synergy* and *Put Your Ears on a Stick,* stated, in looking to future projections, *The humans who will have the competitive differential advantage will be those who develop a balance by allowing technology to enter their worlds, yet control that sometimes uncomfortableness with human touch and concern. Anything that tips the scales too dramatically in one direction too quickly usually has major consequences attached to it.*

In a world with so much black and white, it's important to find the middle ground. John Naisbitt said it best in *Megatrends,*

Whenever institutions introduce new technology to customers or employees, they should build in a high touch component; if they don't, people will try to create their own or reject the new technology. **People must feel they are involved and that their input is not only wanted but also appreciated.**

People planning was made remarkably clear by Al Weber, a consultant to organizations and individuals in the areas of management supervision and sales training. As quoted in *SALON TODAY Management Report,* Weber noted, *You deal on a day-to-day basis with people whose lives have become increasingly complex. The togetherness and sense of belonging we used to share with our family and neighbors is disappearing, and we are looking more to our work environment to satisfy those needs.*

People Participating in Their Futures

Smart salon management knows that people need to be involved in decisions that affect their lives. Greater togetherness within an organization can be achieved by emphasizing an understanding with employees. As noted before, William Ouchi maintains that the success of Japanese growth has come from having each employee experience the specifics of another employee's role. This gives greater respect to each employee's position and stronger comprehension of the organization's overall goals and philosophies.

Ouchi lists some cases where American corporations have adapted the Japanese style to their situation and in general have been successful. It is, however, recognized that while one cannot transpose the entire Japanese system into American business, many components are adaptable. So, progressive salons take the best ideas, involve their people in the planning, and set goals together so that everyone participates in future growth.

Money Planning

A strong emphasis in the salon has and will continue to be in the service aspect of our business. Today however, psy-cosmetologists are sensitive to the importance of having a clear-cut path to their plans and goals. **Formalized salon operating budgets are now recognized as one of the keys to cost-effective spending.** Salons realize that a detailed and workable budget is necessary for sound business principles. Every salon operating expense must be addressed and allotted a specific percentage. These areas are addressed in the money pie, which shows each area in which a traditional salon incurs expenses. Planning expenses can often save money.

THE MONEY PIE

Service Expenses

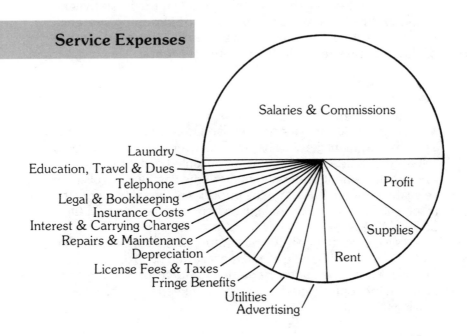

Salaries & Commissions

Laundry
Education, Travel & Dues
Telephone
Legal & Bookkeeping
Insurance Costs
Interest & Carrying Charges
Repairs & Maintenance
Depreciation
License Fees & Taxes
Fringe Benefits
Utilities
Advertising

Profit

Supplies

Rent

Retail Expenses

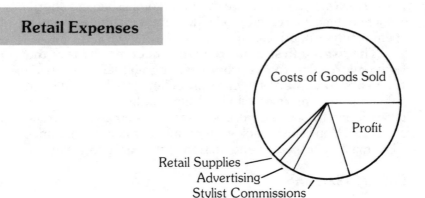

Costs of Goods Sold

Profit

Retail Supplies
Advertising
Stylist Commissions

Successful salons increasingly realize that they have two separate businesses. As the money pie indicates, there is a service business and a retail business. These two areas are often combined; therefore it is sometimes hard to see the true financial picture of the business. It is essential that these two areas be totally separated on the monthly profit and loss statement. **The key is not to have complicated bookkeeping systems, but to have a system that shows clearly a financial picture of the business in both dollars and percents.**

Time Planning

The most important question we can ask you, and to which we unfortunately know the answer, is, "Do you have enough time as an owner, manager, or stylist?" The overwhelming answer is "NO!" We believe time planning can only become successful when management understands that time can be controlled by delegating and refocusing on the priorities of the salon. Often the responsibilities are overwhelming when an owner is a S.M.O.— Stylist, Manager, and Owner.

As we enter the twenty-first century, it is inconceivable that one individual can handle all these areas and do justice to each. The average salon structure is getting too large for one person to maintain the topflight performances that keep a well-oiled salon moving forward.

Finding a Balance

On a daily basis, more owners are delegating responsibilities to the salon staff so that more can be accomplished in a shorter amount of time. Increased productivity frees up time that can be spent on other priorities.

The twenty-first-century owner accepts the fact that being everything to everybody will be virtually useless in the years to come. Time can only be an ally when you're not fighting it from morning till night! One of the resolutions is to diversify and to delegate work, so as to make time a partner, not an enemy! You cannot package time and save it until you want it. Time must be respected and utilized to its fullest potential!

Facility Planning

As we have discussed in early projections, the salons of the future will look and act dramatically different. The physical environment is extremely important to clients. Image making is essential to clients who seek the finest of everything. The salon's image will be designed to attract a particular market by appealing to the specific needs, desires and tastes of the clients in that market. Newness is becoming more and more important to clients. Salons of the future must realize that they cannot just look good on the inside. The outside structure of the salon of the future must have the appeal to draw clients in the front door.

Salons are budgeting for expansion, redesigning, and adding second and third units. Remodeling is essential every five years or less, depending on the clientele. The marketplace is too competitive to have eight- and ten-year-old furniture and equipment.

Clients relate to changes of the physical environment as a statement of growth and prosperity. That's exactly what clients of the twenty-first century want to see and be around. Clients want to go to successful salons, because that's how they're relating to themselves, as successful, ever-growing people. From all indications, salons have picked up this feeling and are addressing this issue in ever-increasing numbers. The sparkling salons of the future will have their doors open to their clientele with the statement going out loud and clear, "We're ready for you!"

The Advertising Game

It is projected that by the twenty-first century, advertising could absorb an average of five percent to ten percent of the existing salon budget. This would make advertising the second or third largest expenditure. For years, salons have been caught in the trap of not having enough monies for advertising or having spent monies in wrong areas of advertising that have not been effective. Hence, they are reluctant to put more good money into what they perceive as a bad return on investment.

Reis and Trout, authors of the book *Positioning: The Battle for Your Mind,* argue that positioning is not only the key word, but the very success of advertising. Clients today and in the future want to be enticed, excited, stimulated, and convinced that you're the one salon that can fulfill their needs. An excerpt from *SALON TODAY Management Report* shows how advertising affects every decision consumers make:

WHY IS IT?

A man wakes up in the morning after sleeping on an advertised bed in advertised pajamas. He will bathe in an advertised tub, wash with advertised soap, shave with an advertised razor, have a breakfast of advertised juice, cereal and toast toasted in an advertised toaster, put on advertised clothes and glance at his advertised watch . . .

He'll ride to work in an advertised car, sit at an advertised desk, smoke advertised cigarettes and write with an advertised pen. Yet this man hesitates to advertise, saying that advertising doesn't pay.

Finally . . . when his business goes under, he'll advertise it for sale. Then it is too late.

WHAT IS IT?

SALON TODAY defines advertising as anything and everything that gets your message across to your regular clients as well as potential new clients.

Remember: Advertising can be as simple and inexpensive as client referrals . . . or as complex and costly as a TV commercial.

The message is clear: No matter if that advertising comes in forms such as direct mail, newspaper, flyers, billboards, magazines, small gift give-aways, public relations, free press, community activity, cut-a-thons, beauty seminars, in-salon promotions, surveys, hair fashion shows, or radio, **the keys are to create interest, stimulate desire, and get clients to react to your advertising. Zero in and direct your advertising to your clients and their needs and success will be yours.**

Planned and Systematic

Advertising is planned and budgeted and is systematic in its functions. The salons of today and the future calculate monies spent, track their investments, and are showing a return on those investments. Because each salon is unique, a form of advertising that is successful under certain circumstances does not necessarily prove productive under others. Salons are coming out of the trial-and-error period and are better prepared to meet the demand for productive and cost-effective advertising. They will not be able to be as competitive in their marketplace and with their existing clientele without that key ingredient called advertising.

Ask Your Clients

Rather than beating your head against a wall about what works and what doesn't work, go to the natural resource that is presently the foundation of your business, your clients. **By surveying clients, you will gain an understanding of who they are and why they frequent your salon.** A cross section of certain information is necessary to establish your findings. For example:

1. What is your age, sex, working status?
2. What services do you require?
3. What other services would you like us to offer?
4. What days and times are most convenient for you to visit our salon?
5. What are the attributes of our salon that attracted you?
6. What areas of our salon do you find least desirable?
7. How many members of your family come here?
8. Do you like to have the option of charging your services and professional products?
9. Do you use coupons you receive in the mail?
10. Do you read a newspaper? Which paper and what sections most interest you?
11. What radio stations do you listen to?
12. Do you belong to a special organization or group within your community?

These questions will start to identify who your clients are and will help make your advertising dollar more profitable.

How Do Clients Find a Salon?

The multitude of research and surveys proves that **client referral is the anchor of salon advertising.** In some instances, client referrals constitute as much as 80 percent of the existing clientele. And yet, as important as that fact is, salons must continue to actively expand their client bases through advertising. In a survey completed by *SALON TODAY Management Report*, the following percentages of salons reported using these forms of advertising:

Public Relations	24%
Newspapers	22%
Direct Mail	13%
Radio	9%
Yellow Pages	9%
In-Salon Promotions	7%
Client Referral Systems	7%
Television	4%
Window Displays	4%
Other	1%

Whatever forms of advertising are used, they must capture the attention of consumers to be effective. Many salons still struggle with advertising, but its importance can no longer be ignored. The fact is clear, **advertising is *imperative* to your salon's growth and success.**

Conclusion

We have come to the end of just some of the trends we perceive as very important to salon growth and success. Trends are issues that affect the four natural resources: people, money, time, and facility. **Recognizing that changes and trends are imminent is basic to the success of the twenty-first century salon.**

We laughed at Buck Rodgers, but Buck is here to stay. With space shuttles and air travel escalating on a daily basis, in the not too distant future, we will develop the first space salon. Many of the projections discussed may not be so futuristic. It is only one's perception that makes a dream a reality.

When colonization does begin, can't we realize that one of the most important leaders will be the psy-cosmetologist of the twenty-second century, or will it be the twenty-first century? Our technology will escalate by leaps and bounds, and our maturing society will benefit from these advancements. However, the essence of the human is the need for love, beauty, and feeling good. The psy-cosmetologist will fulfill those dreams.

The book *Individual Psychology* by Guy J. Manaster and Raymond T. Corsini reflects on how psy-cosmetologists will use their knowledge. Manaster and Corsini say, *Equally important is using knowledge for general human good, permitting people to grow and develop and advance and enhance themselves. Knowledge for the sake of knowledge is fine, but the "use" of knowledge is more important.* **The new psy-cosmetologist will be a leader in our society today and in the future.** These types of individuals will be part of the pioneering spirit needed for the new frontiers of the future.

What will we be doing in the meantime? Well, we have already prebooked our tickets and flight to do the first lecture at the new colony. You see, we believe this seminar is in the not-too-distant future. Oh yes, the name of the seminar is already picked out: Psy-Cosme-Spaceology! See you on the moon! The new psy-cosmetologist is one of the brightest stars in the galaxy! But a different type of star, one that is more interested in making other people shine than in making himself or herself shine.

HIGHLIGHTS FROM CHAPTER 4

Chapter 4 focused on ten trends that will affect the professional salon industry. **Professionals must be constantly aware of the following changes that are occurring in not only their profession, but also in society at large:**

1. Salon professionals who are sensitive to their clients' needs and maintain a positive attitude, project confidence, and cooperate with other team members will have the competitive edge.

2. The salon environment in a high-tech/high-touch age means essentially that the right physical atmosphere targeted to the market will dramatically have an ever-increasing affect on the profession's growth.

3. The better our industry understands the clients' world, the happier and more productive salon professionals will be.

4. The high technology of computerization has graced the professional doorstep. It cannot, and will not, be ignored. The incredible assistance a computer can be to your business is not necessary, but is is the new way to solid profitability.

5. Personal standards within the profession have developed, starting with a code of self-reliance, personal responsibility, and social interest.

6. The changing scope of salon hours is necessary to meet the changing time schedules of the professional clientele. Expanded hours are here, and the time conscious client will go where convenience prevails.

7. The use of telecommunication is the realization that we live in an information age. "Tele-selling" keeps in constant contact with our clients. Telecommunicating expands your market and increases the profitability of the salon.

8. Expanding potential through education has been, and will continue to be, a cornerstone of the profession's growth.

9. Sound management practices that utilize the four natural resources—people, money, time, and facility—will establish a sound business base that will be cost productive and highly profit oriented. Planning, organizing, implementing, and reviewing the business are essential.

10. Advertising is a major key to reaching the customer. Advertising is a year-round investment. The age when a business doesn't advertise has passed by the way. Advertising when you're busy is the secret to very few down times in your business. You can have the best educated salon, but what if no one knows you're there?!

If there would be one trend to put special emphasis on, that would be Trend One: The New Psy-Cosmetologist: A Human Relations Specialist. Psy-cosmetologists' optimum awareness of the sensitive needs of clients is their special strength. The new psy-cosmetologist, with a positive attitude, outward confidence, and a desire to cooperate with team members truly deserves the praise of being called a human relations specialist.

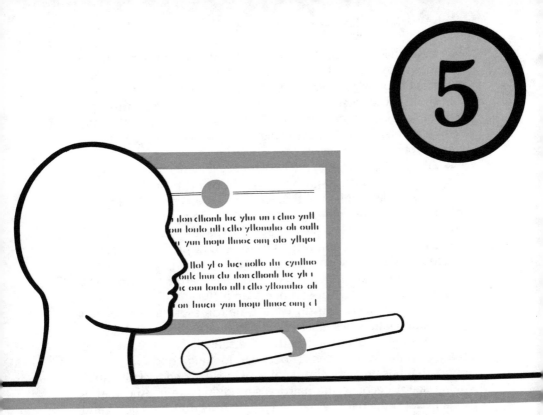

Psy-Cosmetology:
An Idea Whose
Time Has Come

Like children's clothing that no longer fits in their growing and maturing years, the old image of the hairdreser or barber-stylist is becoming increasingly antiquated to the part of society that seeks awareness. After a careful analysis of salons through-out the world, we can say there is clear evidence that many cosmetologists and barber-stylists of today no longer fit the stereotypes of the past.

At social gatherings, the apologetic, self-effacing statement, "I'm just an operator," is giving way to the proud pronouncement, "I'm a hairstylist." It is true that we haven't observed this professional esteem everywhere, but we are seeing much more of it now than we saw only a decade ago. We have seen more college graduates take up shears and combs to become professional artists of people. We have seen clients become much more sensitive to the importance of appearance, and who better to help them achieve their desired appearance than a stylist?

Not everybody can do what a hairdresser can do. It is a profession with skills and talents that are demanded by an ever-sensitive public, and it is this, the sensitivity of the public to the indisputable relationship between looking good and feeling good, that has brought about some of these changes. The public didn't see it because the hairdressers didn't see it. And that is exactly what the hairdresser can help clients do—look good and feel good. How could a profession have lived with such a low image when it had such a high mission? How could such a contribution be minimized, and worse, be taken for granted for so long? We wonder!

Evidence of Change

The evolution of the professional salon industry is occurring today for a variety of reasons. The public is getting greater exposure to the significance of cosmetologists and barber-stylists. Radio, TV talk shows, and newspaper fashion sections are always advertising new cuts, perms, and colors that are advanced by professionals in the industry. The way you get to that style is through the skills of a stylist, and this is not a hard observation for a viewer, listener, or reader to draw.

Almost all models seen on TV or in fashion shows, as well as actors and actresses on the movie screen, were designed by a professional cosmetologist or barber-stylist and a cosmetic specialist. But, as importantly, every neighborhood has salons with less exposure but no less significant contributors to the lives of their clientele.

Besides this increasing exposure that helps upgrade the profession, there is more evidence to support our thesis that the profession is in a positive transition. Consider:

- More and more educational programs today focus on the psychological, communication, and human relations areas. Many barber and beauty schools are training in human relations as well as in technical skills.

- Salons are being run more systematically and are more organized than ever before. The computer has helped larger salons to deal with their records and provide the information to run their businesses more effectively. Even smaller salons are run by owners who are increasingly taking management and communication courses.

- Education and advertising are receiving increasing attention. Many salons have a practice of bringing a consultant from one coast to the other to get an objective view on how to increase profitability and improve communications in their businesses.

- Whereas in 1975 there were two trade magazines supported by the industry, by 1985 there were twice as many information or management reports available.

- Salon personnel are increasingly involved in overall civic and community activities and are taking on responsibilities as community leaders.

- Many well-rounded stylists have chosen to specialize in one or more areas, from perming and coloring to skin care and nails.

- Greater emphasis is being placed on the consultant role of the stylist, to better understand the total needs of the "person" of the client.

- Salons are offering expanded professional services to fulfill clients' wants and needs.

- The overall size of salons has increased to house special services, and staff size has doubled in the decade from 1975 to 1985.

- Salon hours have expanded in response to the needs of working women.

- Salon environments are scientifically and systematically planned and designed for clients' comfort and convenience.

The whispers of these changes become louder the closer you observe this profession. These changes have emerged in response to the Human Revolution occurring in society. We are living in a time when the public is more assertive and educated than ever, and more aware of the fact that *they can choose among professional services*. If one doctor, lawyer, or dentist is not meeting the needs of the 1980s person, another one will. And **if one salon isn't fulfilling the needs of a client, the client will go elsewhere.**

And they do!

Where do they go?

They go where their needs are met.

Who can meet those needs?

Someone who is naturally sensitive to people's changing demands or someone who is formally trained and educated in the psychology of people as well as in the skills of cosmetology.

This is the mission of psy-cosmetology.

This is the message of our book.

BIBLIOGRAPHY

Page

8   Ashley Montagu, *Touching: The Human Significance of Skin* (New York: Harper & Row, 1971), p. 5.

8   Charles Panati, *Breakthroughs* (Boston: Houghton-Mifflin, 1980, pp. 6, 7.

10   John Naisbitt, *Megatrends: Ten New Directions Transforming Our Lives* (New York: Warner Books, 1982).

12   Modern Salon, *1982 Salon Client Survey Summary,* p. 10.

19   George J. Vogel, in personal communication, March, 1984.

25   Thomas J. Peters and Robert Waterman, Jr., *In Search of Excellence* (New York: Harper & Row, 1982), p. 157.

26   Lewis H. Young, "Views on Management" (speech to Ward Howell International, Links Club, New York, Dec. 2, 1980), p. 5.

37   Lewis E. Losoncy, *Innovative Psychotherapies* (New York: Wiley Interscience, 1982), p. 286.

66   Joshua Liebman, *Hope for Man* (New York: Simon & Schuster, 1966.

86   William Ouchi, *Theory Z* Reading, Massachusetts: Adeson Wesley, 1981).

118   Christopher C. Reilly, "Salon Synergy" (seminar, Philadelphia, Pennsylvania, April 11, 1983).

119   John Naisbitt, *Megatrends* (New York: Warner Books, 1982), p. 43.

119   Al Weber, "Ten Ways to Motivate Your Employees," *SALON TODAY International Management Report,* Vol. 1 No. 2, 1983, p. 7.

122   Al Reis and Jack Trout, *Positioning: The Battle for Your Mind* (New York: Warner Books, 1982).

122   "Why Is It?" *SALON TODAY,* Vol. 1 No. 3, 1983, p. 3.

123   "What Is It?" *SALON TODAY,* Vol. 1 No. 3, 1983, p. 3.

124   "Prized Promos" *SALON TODAY,* Vol. 1 No. 3, 1983, p. 3.

125   Raymond T. Corsini and Guy J. Manaster, *Individual Psychology* (Itasca, Illinois: F. E. Peacock, 1982), p.7.

ACKNOWLEDGEMENTS

This book is only a reflection of what we observed in the cosmetology and barber-styling professions. We are not the creators of The New Psy-Cosmetologists, but are only the reporters. The true acknowledgements go to the hundreds of thousands of caring professionals who were psy-cosmetologists long before we created the term. So, this book is dedicated to every caring hair, skin or nail professional who realizes that it's not just *how they cut,* but *who they are.*

So many people deserve credit for this book, and even more importantly, credit for uplifting the beauty and barbering professions. We salute those tens of thousands of salon owners and managers who motivated their people to feel pride and growth that only further education can give. They were the true people developers. A thanks to the many manufacturers and distributors and their sales consultants who made a commitment to educating their salon accounts and developed the guest artists who gave up their weekends to share their expertise.

We particularly thank Deborah Youmans, who took a risk, and for the first time ever, took psy-cosmetology to the public at the Des Moines Civic Center. A special acknowledgement is also due to the first group of psy-cosmetologists who showed their dedication to professional and personal growth by attending the first formal psy-cosmetology training workshop in Reading, Pennsylvania.

To all of those hair professionals who have shared their feelings, desires, and most importantly, their advice, we thank them for their courage in speaking out. We hope that this book fills their caring expectations. And congratulations especially to every single hairstylist who, instead of staying home on a Sunday or Monday, drove miles to educational events to learn more about cosmetology, business, advertising, . . . and psychology. It is because of the efforts at each of these levels multiplied over and over again each weekend that we see a profession in dramatic transition.

More than anyone else, Howard Hafetz, our friend and inspiration, deserves the credit for this book. We know of no other person who believed in the importance of upgrading the cosmetology and barber-styling professions more than Howard Hafetz, President of one of America's leading full-service beauty supply distributorships.

Howard believed that the road to professionalism was education, which not only brought knowledge, but self-respect, pride, and greater fulfillment. He tread onward despite cries from small thinkers who said, "Hairdressers don't care about education." Only we co-authors know how many major decisions Howard made based on selfless motives to professionalize the salon industry.

Howard brought us co-authors together. He encouraged us when we were down. He published this book despite pressures not to by others who thought they had a monopoly on helping. Yes, Howard, while most will never realize your sacrifices to make education as important as shears and combs, we saw. You are the true author of *The New Psy-Cosmetologist*.

We also thank Joe Tammaro, perhaps the top educational media expert in the industry, for putting together our educational program in psy-cosmetology at the International Institute. Joe can take an idea and, through the use of media, bring it to life and flow into the minds and hearts of the participants.

Vicki Christopher, Publisher of *SALON TODAY Management Report,* worked with obsession to provide opportunities for us to work simply everywhere to get a true cross-section of what was happening within the profession. Her efforts resulted in our broad experience, without which we could not have written this book. Thanks, Vicki.

Karen Miller-Garrett, Editor of *SALON TODAY* and Lew Losoncy's former student, from whom he now learns, faced unbelievable demands to complete this project with not one complaint. It could not have happened in the same way without her.

To all of the people at *SALON TODAY,* especially Betsy Reinhart who typed the first and second manuscripts. Betsy will never know how important she was.

A special thanks to the artists of The Main Idea advertising agency—Marie Gernert, Sheryl Dusel, Pam Ries, and Penny Hammond—for their creative design of this book.

And our sincere appreciation to Gary Lyons for sharing his expertise and guidance in helping us publish our work.

Personal Acknowledgements
From Donald Scoleri

To my wife Joan, for without her love, support and constant encouragement, my co-authorship would not have become a reality. Her constant retyping of the book late at night so I could see a finished page in the morning was deeply appreciated.

To my children, Donna and Charles, for their understanding and love when Dad is often away while other fathers are home. They are my special inner strength.

To Anthony and Carmella Scoleri, my parents, who have always been by my side through the good times and the bad times—especially in the bad times. No parents have given more love to children, family and friends like Carmella and Anthony Scoleri.

To my brother Anthony, who has taught me that action and deeds speak louder than words. His support to "go for it" was always in my mind while writing this book.

To Joe Tammaro, my mentor, friend, partner, and confidante, who always made me believe that I was capable of attaining any goal if I believed in myself. Joe has the insightful ability to see what humans are capable of, and then a little more.

Finally, to Lew Losoncy, his new bride Pam, and their daughter Shauna, Lew Losoncy encouraged me as a first-time author to believe in my words and put them into print for the world to read.

Personal Acknowledgements
From Lew Losoncy

Specifically, I wish to acknowledge the most important person in my life, my wife and friend and a true psy-cosmetologist herself—Pam. Whenever I strayed one inch from the deep understandings of what a psy-cosmetologist was, Pam was determined to keep me on course. Little Shauna, as well, rounded out our team as she showed me how not to be afraid to explore new learnings and express what I felt.

To my friend Steve Cowan, a solid citizen who believed. And to my partner, Donald, whose friendship and sensitivity for his co-professionals made this book have not just words, but *feelings*.

ABOUT THE AUTHORS

Dr. Lewis E. Losoncy is a psychologist, international educator, and author of several best-selling books including *Turning People On, You Can Do It,* and *The Motivating Leader.* He has lectured in many industries, businesses and schools on the topics of motivation and encouragement.

Dr. Lew has worked with salons in 48 of the United States, most of the Canadian Provinces, as well as Australia and New Zealand. More than any other non-cosmetologist, Dr. Losoncy has made significant progress in helping the public realize the valuable contribution of salon professionals in our society.

A former college professor, Dr. Losoncy earned his Doctorate in human development at Lehigh University in Bethlehem, Pennsylvania, and presently serves on the faculty of the International Institute for the Study of Psy-Cosmetology in Reading, Pennsylvania. Like many authors, Dr. Lew enjoys working in the serene setting of his home by the ocean. He lives with his wife Pam and daughter Shauna on Long Beach Island in New Jersey.

Donald W. Scoleri, cosmetologist and national educator, is considered by many to be the most practical human communication and salon management expert in the industry. He has become an inspirational leader among salon professionals through his work at *every* level of the salon business—from stylist and colorist to salon manager/owner, to management positions at both distribution and manufacturing levels.

Donald has lectured in 47 of the United States and all of the Canadian Provinces. His warm way with people and his grass-roots knowledge of everyday salon experiences have won Donald the hearts of his peers as well as thousands of salon professionals who have benefited from his expertise.

Through his extensive travels as a lecturer, Donald has come to feel at home anywhere in America. But, he feels *most* at home when with his wife Joan and their children, Donna and Charles, at their residence in Berlin, New Jersey.